STRENGTH
OF HEART

JUDY A. FREDETTE

STRENGTH OF HEART

An Optimistic Journey Through Breast Cancer

iUniverse, Inc.
Bloomington

STRENGTH OF HEART
AN OPTIMISTIC JOURNEY THROUGH BREAST CANCER

iUniverse books may be ordered through booksellers or by contacting:

iUniverse
1663 Liberty Drive
Bloomington, IN 47403
www.iuniverse.com
1-800-Authors (1-800-288-4677)

ISBN: 978-1-4759-0550-2 (sc)
ISBN: 978-1-4759-0551-9 (ebk)

Printed in the United States of America

iUniverse rev. date: 03/27/2012

My story is dedicated with love, to my daughters: Heidi, Heather & Aimee; and my granddaughters: Jocelyn, Ivy, and Zariah. You have brought such joy into my life. My hope is that a cure for cancer will be discovered in your lifetimes!

I would like to extend my most sincere appreciation to... God, my family & friends, my physicians and nurses ,my fellow cancer survivors, and the MWCC RN Class of 2011... it is because of all of you that I have survived! ☺

Special acknowledgement and appreciation to Sarah (for editing), to Heather (for proofreading), and to Brett (for suggesting the title of this book). Thank you!

DIAGNOSIS & SURGERY

I'm not sure where to begin . . . or when telling a story like this if it even matters where I begin . . . but with all stories, there must be a beginning. I grew up knowing someday I may get diabetes. My mother had been diagnosed with Type II diabetes when I was in nursing school and she died from complications of the disease thirty years later. I knew that heart disease was a possibility . . . my maternal grandfather and uncles had died from heart disease. I knew enough to be careful with alcohol . . . my father had died when I was merely thirteen of cirrhosis of the liver. I knew I would face a constant battle with obesity since I came from a family of obese women. But cancer . . . I thought I was immune. I never worried about it. I never thought about it.

I was living my life, having a family, furthering my education, working, surviving like most anyone else does. I have been blessed with many friendships and a loving family, many who have been critical to my recovery. It is important for me to share some thoughts about each of them. My husband Brian and I have been together for over thirty years of our lives. How many girls get to marry the cutest boy in fourth grade? I can remember begging our babysitter to take us for walks by his house. I would also say my prayers that I would marry Brian Fredette one day . . . but I was also praying to be able to wear a bra! Just goes to show you that one must be very careful about what they pray for! God does have a sense of humor. Our daughters have always enjoyed these stories. Of course, we didn't start dating and committing to spend our lives together until much later. One summer day when my girlfriend and I were driving around, as was popular in those days, she insisted that we stop to talk to Brian and his friend Tom. I think she was interested in Brian. I know now that it was my good fortune, when he talked past my friend to ask me out on a date, and from there our story as a couple begins. We've had the ups and downs as most marriages do but honestly, I can't think of a better person to share my life with. I've always told our daughters to choose the man who would be sitting with you one day holding your hand and encouraging you when you are sick. My advice held true.

Let me tell you about our oldest daughter, Heidi. Heidi has always had an easy-going, adventurous personality. Her philosophy was that life is a party and everyday should be a good day. She moved to California when she graduated from college. We told her not to fall in love and have our grandbabies out there . . . well she did so anyhow. She fell in love with Ainsley and together they have a beautiful daughter, Ivy Rose. I believe that motherhood has changed her life philosophy somewhat. However, I am very sure that she will be a really fun mother. Her spirit has always reminded me of my own mother. Although she is distanced from our immediate family by miles, the technology of today keeps us connected.

Heather is our middle child. And anyone who knows about middle children, she has all of those qualities. She is our worrier and has always been the one to make sure that our family is "okay." She is a reading specialist and takes this role very seriously. Heather is always there for her family and others. She really gives so much. She is engaged (finally after six years!) to her soul-mate Corey, and will be getting married in a destination wedding next month.

Aimee is our most practical daughter. She has faced some interesting challenges in life, and because of the love of her family has come out ahead. She is a cardiac nurse by career, working the night shift. She is engaged to a good man, Chris. I knew Chris was a good man when for Aimee's birthday eight months after my diagnosis, he handed me a wrapped package. Inside was a necklace with a silver "survivor" charm on it. Together they have two beautiful daughters, Jocelyn and Zariah, just thirteen months apart. I can remember Aimee saying once that she had her sisters all figured out . . ." Heidi likes to party too much, and Heather needs to

2

party more." Times have changed their priorities now and partying takes on new meaning. Because she is the nurse and the practical one, she has been chosen to be our health care proxy.

I have two younger siblings, Janice and Barry. He has three children and two grandchildren. He just lives in the next town but we don't see each other as often as I would like. However, it is comforting to know that if I needed him he would be there for me. My sister Janice has been married to the same man, Ken since she was sixteen years old. Their love is deep and together they have seven children and recently a grandson. As sisters often are, Janice and I are close and support each other in so many ways.

Renee is Brian's sister, therefore my sister-in-law. Renee is a person I would choose as a friend even if we were not related. She and her husband, Pat, are the proud parents of a rat terrier, Mabel and a boston terrier, Mary. They are a fun couple to be around. Some of our favorite travel stories include Renee and Pat.

Bob and Gloria are Brian's parents. For years they would talk about retiring and now that they are retired, their lives are busier than ever. When my mother died, Bob told me that they would take care of me and for me not to worry. I reminded them of this when I was first diagnosed. I needed them more than ever. They didn't try to replace my mother but offered what they could for me. And they were there for me, which I will always be grateful for.

Paula and Jim are our very best friends. We became friends when our children were very little. It all started with a game of pitch and some "cheap" chips. We had brought the chips (not cheap) to their house to play cards. Jim thought Paula bought them and complained about the "cheap chips", a brand that he did not like. You can imagine his face when he learned that the new friends had brought them. So even after that we have continued to come back over the years and our friendship has grown. Certainly you have heard the saying that friends are the family you choose for yourself . . . and we did choose them! The joys and sorrows of life have been shared and easier to bear with the connection between our families.

Brian and I have never really had empty nest syndrome. We have two Italian Greyhound dogs who have been members of our families for many years now. They are old girls now with Daisy at age fifteen in dog-years and Angel at age ten in dog-years. They "worked" very hard during my journey to "nurse" me back to healthy. And although it may have seemed like they were just lying on the couch with me, the warmth of their love comforted me during many sad days.

I had my annual physicals and routine screenings, but only because I am a "rule follower" and those were the guidelines for good health. I never expected what was to come. I am a professor of nursing at a small community college and classes had just started. It was a busy time so I had rescheduled my mammogram to the following week. I can remember laughing with colleagues as we shared our common dislike of mammograms.

For many years I worked as a nurse in the hospital where I received and trusted my healthcare. Employees knew me. As I waited in the mammogram room for the technician to review my digital films for clarity, I reminded her to check my right breast since they had been "watching" a spot on that breast. "You mean your left" she replied. "No" I said, "definitely my right." "Oh no," was her response and this is where my story really begins.

"Okay, so there is something on my left breast" . . . I can remember thinking. "No problem, they will just watch it like they have been the right". I scheduled an ultrasound of my left breast as recommended by the radiologist before leaving that day. Two days later while having the ultrasound, more concern was expressed by the professionals involved and a biopsy was suggested.

Fortunately, I was able to schedule the biopsy right after the Columbus Day weekend. I never knew that three days could feel like three months, or three years. Breast biopsies at this hospital are done in the ultrasound room. I was prepared, draped and had the procedure explained to me. The physician performing the biopsy was known to me, not as well then as she would be in the future. I can remember her saying to me that "she knew all about breast cancer". Of course she did, I thought. I trusted her. She went on to explain to me she had breast cancer two years prior. I was not sure how that was possible because she looked so good. She was smiling and positive. She went on to explain to me that she does not share personal information with just anyone. I felt comforted by her words.

Specimens were collected and I changed into my street clothes. I asked how it looked and actually pleaded to know more about what was to come. I asked for honesty. The physician said it did not look good but that we needed to wait for the specimen to be tested. I can remember thinking how lucky I was that my best friend was the manager in the histology department. I was hoping for my specimen diagnosis to be expedited. I left the room feeling scared but composed. Or I thought I was. The more I walked toward the hospital exit, the more I cried. I felt so vulnerable.

As I walked toward the hospital exit, I looked down the hallway to the oncology department. Dr. D's office door was open. I had always liked Dr. D. and had a nice working relationship with her. She was knowledgeable and respected by many patients and professionals. My decision was spontaneous and down I walked into her office. I can remember her looking up at me, a bowl of soup in front of her and a spoon in her hand. This was likely her first "quiet" moment of the day and now she had this hysterical woman in front of her. I told her there was a lump in my breast and if it was cancer I wanted her to be my doctor. She very calmly told me that if it is cancer that we would get through it.

She said "we" . . . that must mean she will be my doctor I thought. I walked out of the hospital that day thinking I had a plan. A plan I hoped I would not be executed but at least it was in place.

Two days later, I phoned the histology department for my results. I was sitting at my desk at work. It was October 15th. It was my oldest daughter's birthday. I can remember just hoping I didn't have to share bad news with her on this special day. The phone rang and rang. Finally someone answered and my best friend had to tell her best friend she had cancer. She later told me it was the most difficult thing she ever had to do. However, I was glad it was her that told me. I knew she cared about me because for some reason it was a bit less painful to hear it from someone who cares about you. It was still cancer but it seemed different. I can remember setting the phone down and wondering what to do next.

I picked the phone back up minutes later and called my friend Tina who is a nurse practitioner. A nurse practitioner who just happens to work closely with Dr. D. I told her I had breast cancer and that I didn't know what to do. She told me I would be alright and she would be with me every step of the way. Just hearing her voice made me feel better. I was not sure if I believed her, but I did feel better momentarily. I tried to continue working but it was impossible, so I headed home. On the way, I called my husband, Brian. There was an uncomfortable silence on the other end. He finally spoke and shared his thoughts that he had convinced himself all would be fine with me. He was shocked but assured me we would get through it. Again, hearing his voice made me feel better but I still was not convinced I would be okay.

Sleep did not come easily that night. I can remember thinking that sleep, or lack of, would likely be a problem in the coming weeks and months, if I were to make it that long. The next day, I went to the hospital to see a few friends and colleagues, hoping as I shared my diagnosis that somebody might have some encouraging words for me. I was ready to share with anyone who would listen. I can remember being at the elevator when a colleague asked how I was doing. I turned to her and told her I had breast cancer. "I think I'm going to puke" was her response. At the time, I can remember thinking her response was not very supportive. She later emailed an apology explaining she was shocked by what I had said and she didn't know how a nice person like me could get cancer. The reality is that cancer does not discriminate . . . there is an equal opportunity for all.

The next day, I shared my diagnosis with my nursing students. I was conflicted with this decision, but the teacher in me decided someone may as well learn from my experience. Something good could come from something bad. I stood before the class of sixty students and told them the truth. I encouraged them to ask any questions at any time. The reaction from my students varied . . . some cried, some sat in disbelief, some came to hug me, some prayed, but all expressed to me they were grateful I shared my diagnosis with them. That same day, and in the weeks that followed, several beautiful women, Chris, Shelley, Laura, Kathie, Linda, Ann, and Anita, shared their breast cancer survival stories with me. For two days I had been dying, but now I knew I would live. By sharing their stories I was empowered to survive. My hope is that I might do the same for others as they did for me. And now my story continues through my email updates sent to family, friends, and students. I shared with anyone who would listen as well as anyone who wanted to receive my emails. I took pictures along the way, all the while thinking someday I would be happy I did . . . and hoping I would live to see that someday. I suddenly had another reason to fight harder.

*   *   *

October 17, 2009

Dear Family & Friends,

I am writing to share some very upsetting news. I was diagnosed with breast cancer on Thursday. It was caught on a routine mammogram last week. My best friend who is the manager in histology was the one who had to give me the histology results which must have been horribly painful for her. But all is not doom and gloom . . . I have an appointment at Mass General's Breast Cancer Center for this coming Wednesday. I will see an interdisciplinary team consisting of a breast surgeon, a plastic surgeon, an internist, an oncologist and a radiologist. The appointment will last 3-5 hours. The team will discuss my case and present options to me.

I have absolutely no family history of cancer. My theory is that stress triggered all of this. We know it can happen and for me it did. I've been researching the concept. There was a study done in Scandenavia which showed that women experiencing more than one month of intense stress have twice the likelihood of getting breast cancer.

I'm working on keeping positive . . . I can actually feel all the love and support around me. Please keep me in your prayers and share with any praying people you know. I believe in the power of prayer and positive thoughts. In fact, if you know of any prayer lines/ groups please add my name and cause . . . denomination doesn't matter . . . they all go to the same place!

Love,
Judy

P.S. For my PhD classmates, so sorry to share this by email but I wanted you to know ASAP. I have shared with our professor but felt it would be too difficult to tell you in class. My plan is to continue to keep my life as normal as possible for as long as I can.

* * *

October 21, 2009

Dear Family & Friends,

What a day! What a day filled with hope and love . . . this is because of all of you . . . your prayers and positive thoughts were/are with me . . . I could feel it this afternoon and continue to feel it as I write this update!

Brian and Janice went with me. There was a minor problem when 30 miles from Mass General I realized that I had forgotten my mammogram films. I practically had a meltdown . . . My in-laws saved the day though . . . thank you again Bob & Gloria! Brian and Janice dropped me off, took the red line to Alwife to meet Bob and Gloria,

8

and returned within the hour! Fortunately it did not hold things up . . . without those films I would have had to reschedule.

Mass General's Breast Cancer Center is so wonderful. They were friendly, encouraging and organized. I met with the radiologist, medical assistant, nurse practitioner, clinic manager and breast surgeon. After reviewing my case the team said that it appears to be Stage 1 and very small. I was a bit disappointed to learn that my estrogen receptor test was negative but Dr. G. believes that it is more important that the mass is small and Stage 1. So to me this sounds like more good news!

The plan at this point is that I will have a lumpectomy. I still need to phone tomorrow for a date and will arrange it as soon as possible. I want this foreign invader OUT of my body! During the lumpectomy my axillary lymph nodes will be checked in pathology while I am still in the operating room. Best case scenario, if the nodes are negative then I will have six weeks of daily radiation. The surgery would only be five hours and I would go home the same day with one week out of work. If the nodes are positive, I will likely need chemo followed by radiation needing more time off from work. The experts have advised me that a lumpectomy with radiation has the same results as a mastectomy. I am satisfied and encouraged with this plan. I will have the surgery in Boston and follow-up with Dr. D. locally for chemo and/or radiation.

I will send you the date of surgery when I know. Please keep your prayers and positive thoughts coming my way. And please know how much I love you all!

Take care,
Judy

*   *   *

October 22, 2009

Dear Family & Friends,

I have a surgery date . . . November 12th. I would have liked it sooner but I must remember that Judy Fredette is not the only woman with breast cancer. I must wait my turn. So while I wait I will work on losing some weight and exercising . . . this is what I can do to make a difference. Dr. D. says that there are correlations between obesity and breast cancer. And it is something that I can control . . .

Please continue to keep me in your thoughts and prayers . . . . the wait is so difficult.

Love,
Judy

*   *   *

October 29, 2009

Hello Friends and Family,

Just a quick update . . . the wait seems so long. Two weeks from today will be my surgery.

I'm just so anxious to know my plan. It's hard to be the patient . . . when I'm the nurse I have much more control! Can you believe I actually phoned MGH today to see if they've had any cancellations?

For the most part I am doing fine. I've been walking every "dry" day. Lily (my youngest daughter Aimee's Italian Greyhound puppy) has been a great walking partner. She seems to put a smile on everyone's face, including my own. I've made many new friends on our walks. I'm eating more veggies although I thought I might be allergic. My colleagues assure me that I'm not. I've also had both my seasonal and H1N1 flu shots. I also made an appointment for a physical with my PCP for next week. I will definitely be ready for November 12th!

Our local newspaper had an article yesterday about breast cancer . . . my only risk factor was obesity. So any of you in my category, please get walking too! I was very encouraged to read about the advances that have been made with breast cancer. There was another article today about Dr. and Mrs. M's daughter, T. She fought a breast cancer battle and won. Perhaps one day there will be an article about me!

Please keep those positive thoughts and prayers coming my way . . .

Love,
Judy

* * *

November 5, 2009

Hello Family & Friends,

One more week . . . well hopefully one more week. I just received an upsetting voicemail message from the hospital saying that I missed a mammogram appointment on 10/30 and that they might have to delay my surgery. I knew nothing of this appointment and have actually spoken to two people in that office this week and no mention of it. I have been hypervigilent about all of this and would never have missed an appointment. I will phone them tomorrow to try to straighten this out but right now I am very upset.

On a lighter note, I enjoyed a girls night earlier where my daughters Heather & Aimee, Renee (my sister-in-law) and my mother-in-law, Gloria went for a manicure and pedicure. We all have pink toes with a pink ribbon on our great toes! They are very stylish . . . the manicurists tell me that they will paint their toes in a similar fashion to honor me and other women fighting this battle! We may have started a trend . . .

A colleague friend of mine told me last week that she thinks that all of this may be happening to me for me to realize all the people who love and care for me. I must tell you that I have always felt loved and cared for by all of you . . . but even more so now. Thank you all for loving me and caring so much. Let's keep on with our plan to have some answers on the 12th . . . I'll keep you updated.

Love,
Judy

*   *   *

November 6, 2009

Hello All . . . The hospital coordinator admitted it was her fault, apologized, I forgave her, she booked a mammogram in Boston for Monday, surgery still scheduled for Thursday, so I'm back on track . . . Love, Judy

*   *   *

November 10, 2009

Dear Family & Friends,

Well, some more good news . . . and I KNOW it is because of all the prayers and positive energy coming my way from all of you. I went to MGH yesterday for a 2 ½ hour appointment for multiple mammogram films to prepare for Thursday's surgery. The appointment went well . . . although I did get into a bit of trouble when I asked the mammogram tech if her lovely accent was from England or Australia . . . oops, she was Irish!!! Perhaps that is why my appointment took so long! But the good news is . . . that the cancer is still the same size while I've been waiting for surgery.

Can you believe that in less than 48 hours the cancer will be removed from my body? And in less than 48 hours I will know what my plan for recovery will involve? I must share with you what my morning of surgery will be like . . . a visual to go along with all those positive thoughts and prayers! Well,

first I am to take Ativan 1mg to relax me,
second I will apply a Scopolomine patch to
the back of my ear so I don't get car sick or
sick from anesthesia . . . and then I must
rub Emla cream (numbing cream) all over
my left breast and then wrap it (yes, my left
breast) in saran wrap!!! It is MGH so the
nurse in me knows that this all makes sense,
but I can't help but wonder if my sense of
humor is being tested. I'll have to remember
to send Brian tomorrow to pick up the Saran
wrap . . . hopefully there are enough rolls on
the shelf!

So as you can see I am keeping in good
spirits but I must admit that I am a bit
anxious. I feel the anxiety about the surgery
itself (or the prep for surgery!) but I know I
will be okay. And I know that because of all
of the love and support from all of you. Thank
you! Thank you! Thank you!

Love,
Judy

P.S. Please don't worry if you don't get an
email until Friday morning as we're not sure
what time we will return from the hospital.
I will be in good hands . . . Brian, Heather
and Aimee will be with me . . . and of course
all of you will also be with me in spirit!

*   *   *

It was so difficult for me the day before surgery. I worked with
my students in the clinical setting in the morning. In the afternoon
we went to an off-site conference room for the students to do their
teaching project presentations. At the end of the afternoon, one of
the students, an African-American male student, stood up. It was

dark outside and quiet in our surroundings. He asked for the group to stand, join hands and pray the *Our Father* for me . . . to give me strength, hope, love, and courage. I still wonder to this day if he realizes how much those words meant to me.

That evening friends came to visit me, two teen girls and their mother, a breast cancer survivor. They brought with them a "lucky" breast cancer bear and lots of love and hope. I did bring the bear to surgery with me and to all of my treatments. It has been passed on now to another friend who was recently diagnosed with breast cancer at age 36. Another visitor that evening was my very best friend Paula. I knew she would come. And she came with a beautiful hand-made quilt with the breast cancer ribbon in the pattern. It is beautiful and continues to wrap me with warmth and love.

At this point in my journey, I had already learned so much about breast cancer and was sharing with anyone who would listen to me . . .

- Only 10-20% of breast cancer patients have a family history.
- Infiltrating ductal carcinoma is the most common.
- For most it is the left breast that is affected.
- It is very scary.
- Breast cancer sucks.
- There is a link between obesity and breast cancer.
- Most women with breast cancer do survive.
- Oncotype is only used in ER (estrogen receptor) positive patients. It is not approved for predicting outcomes in ER negative patients.
- Blue dye or isotope is injected for detection of sentinel node.
- MGH Breast Clinic is wonderful
- Chemo if needed would start 2-3 weeks after surgery or later depending on healing.
- I am not alone, I am loved, and I will survive!

Family, friends and colleagues were sending me emails and cards with words of encouragement. I actually took pictures of every card and made it into an album. When I was feeling sad and discouraged, I would reread the messages of hope, support and love that had been sent to me. I still read them sometimes. Their words would energize me with hope, faith and motivation. I desperately needed this support and looked forward to it. A friend sent me these well-known words from an unknown author. I lived by them during my journey and will continue to believe these words forever.

What Cancer Cannot Do

It cannot cripple Love, It cannot shatter Hope, It cannot corrode Faith, It cannot destroy Peace, It cannot kill Friendship, It cannot suppress Memories, It cannot silence Courage, It cannot invade the Soul, It cannot steal Eternal Life, It cannot conquer the Spirit.

One friend gave me a medal blessed by the Pope and another friend sent me this prayer often said before surgery:

Heavenly Father, caring and compassionate God, You never fail to help those who call on You. Give me courage and strength in my hour of need. Guide the doctors who are diagnosing my illness. Assist the surgeons and staff during surgery. Help all those who will care for me. Give them patience and the virtues they need to assist me. Hold me, Divine Physician, in the palm of Your hand where I always will be safe from harm. Trusting in your protection, I shall overcome my fears, for You are always with me. Amen.

My students played such a supporting role in my journey. One of my clinical groups, a group of six fine young women . . . who are now fine young nurses . . . gave me a pearl necklace of faith, courage, and hope. Inside the card they had this story of "The Pearl". I do not know the author . . .

When an oyster is hit with a trauma-a foreign body that invades its' sheltered life, it lives in its' safe shell, it takes action. It builds upon that painful intrusion in its life, adding layer upon layer of iridescence until it creates a pearl-an object valued for its' depth of beauty. The pearl is the beautiful hope born out of the oysters' pain. Just like the pearl, we can be inspired to take action in our own lives to create beauty and hope out of times that are traumatic and painful. We can create something strong that will be admired by all we let see it, for the depth of its' many layers-the beauty of its strength. We can transform what life brings us and use it to move forward with wisdom and grace.

* * *

November 12, 2009

Dear Family & Friends!

Wow, I am overwhelmed by all of the love and support I have felt today. Our prayers have been answered. Just a quick note to let you know that the nodes were NEGATIVE! YIPPPEEE! The "true" report will not come back for 9 days but is rarely different I am told. I will send more information this weekend . . . tonight I am exhausted and medicated. Thank you all for being with me on this journey! I truly couldn't do it without all of you.

Love,
Judy

* * *

November 21, 2009

Hello All . . . Just a very quick update to let you know that Dr. G., my breast surgeon, called this morning. The pathology report just came back. The tumor was 1.3 cm, all margins are clear, and the sentinel node was negative. This is all such wonderful news! Dr. D., my oncologist, will review the report on Monday and discuss the treatment plan with me. I'll share more as soon as I know! Thank you for supporting me through this journey. Enjoy your weekend! Love, Judy

* * *

November 23, 2009

Hello Family & Friends,

I just heard from Dr. D. Because I am estrogen receptor negative and can't receive Tamoxifen for 5 years post cancer, I will have to have chemotherapy now. I was hoping that it would not be necessary but the nurse in me understands why it is very necessary. I will admit that I am not happy about it . . . but I will be happy knowing that it will decrease the risk of the cancer ever coming back! And I do still have all of you by my side so this is the time to do it. The plan is for chemotherapy once every two weeks for eight weeks then once weekly for four weeks. The reality is that I will lose my hair but it is only hair (as I must keep reminding myself) . . . But now I can test out the theory to see if "bald really is beautiful!" My first treatment is Monday 11/30 . . .

So as we approach this Thanksgiving holiday . . . please know that I am thankful that our prayers were answered and that the margins are clear and that the nodes are negative. But most of all I am very thankful to be loved and cared for by all of you! Please know how grateful I am and will always be to have you all in my life!

Love,
Judy

*   *   *

Learning I would need chemotherapy was much more difficult for me than expected and much more upsetting than I shared with others. In my upset I reached out to the women who had originally given me hope. I asked for their advice and this is what they shared with me.

Nora (newly diagnosed and in treatment): "The Cytoxan is the drug that makes your hair fallout. I had 4 drip bags each time-Benadryl, Decadron (reduces fluid retention) and the 2 chemo drugs-Taxatare and Cytoxan. Laugh and joke a lot Judy . . . it really helps! Your hair loss will start 12-14 days after 1st chemo treatment. As soon as it starts, shave. Don't delay-it's too traumatic. Go get your wig now! Go with your own hair so they can see what you want to look like. You can be matched so close that nobody will even know that you are wearing a wig. Decadron (if you have this one) will make you very hyper. I had trouble sleeping. Have someone sit with you through each treatment-that helps too. It is possible that you could end up with a metallic taste in your mouth. Constipation is a huge problem with these drugs. Prepare yourself before and after each treatment. I will keep sending more advice as I think of stuff. You'll be OK Judy. Fight like a girl!"

Barbara (a nurse & 2 year breast cancer survivor): "Things are moving swiftly for you. I remember clearly how I was terrified to go the first day of chemo. I imagined it would hurt and I would be sick right away and that was not so. I had T/C also, with decadron, the steroids also made me way hyper but I didn't fight it. I just stayed up really late and cleaned and was productive. As soon as I started my chemo I went to find a wig. Then when my hair started to fall out, I invited my friend over (who was also hairless due to chemo) and we had some drinks and shaved my head! There were a lot of tears and a lot of laughter that night. Doing it this way made me feel like I had some control in this scary time. I let my friends know when I would be in for chemo and asked for them to visit me on the oncology unit. I also brought a bag along filled with books, magazines, candy, etc. in case I needed to be busy. I didn't really use it but it felt good to have it there, in case. Plan on resting/sleeping chemo week. It is very exhausting for our bodies. Don't make plans/commitments, everything can wait, while you take care of yourself and rest! Note that some people get a lot of hip/joint/bone pain a few days after the Neulasta. When I felt it I was terrified because nobody had explained it to me. I hope it doesn't happen to you. Judy, we are strong women, we do what we have to. You will be alright! We are here for you."

Kathie (a pharmacist & 7 year breast cancer survivor): "Don't be afraid. You will be taken care of by some wonderful people. Believe it or not the chemo is a little anticlimactic. You really won't notice anything on infusion day other than be prepared to pee bright red. The Adriamycin comes out the same color it goes in. The premedication is very effective. You won't notice anything really until 3-4 days later. Being tired is an unusual sensation. It's more like an exhaustion that even sleep won't cure. I won't lie. The AC is hard. Allow yourself a few days each cycle to recover. Mostly it's the fatigue that gets to you. You will have some steroids for premedication and these will keep you in a bright mood for the first 2-3 days. As they wear off the fatigue kicks in about the same time. Plan for lighter activity on these days. But it passes as well. The fatigue wears off and then you do get a few normal days before the next cycle."

Chris (a college professor currently in treatment for breast cancer): "Each infusion is a major step in your journey back to good health. And after chemotherapy, six weeks of radiation is a "piece of cake"! Be prepared for the bone crushing fatigue, it is unbelievable! I would recommend *Biotene* mouthwash for dry mouth because it is often a side effect from the chemotherapy. And a stool softener would also be good to prevent constipation which is another side effect. This is a tough time, Judy. Give in to the fatigue and rest. Keep in mind that it is just temporary and will be behind you soon. Hang in there . . . I am thinking of you often. Try to enjoy life even if you are not feeling like your usual self! It's like belonging to an elite club . . . but not one that you really want to belong to."

Marilyn (a nurse, physician's wife and 13 year breast cancer survivor whose daughter is also a breast cancer survivor): "I think it's great that you are starting your chemotherapy so soon. The more time we all spend thinking and worrying the worse we are so let's get the show on the road. You've had wonderful support and I have little to add except: BE A QUEEN. Do things if and when you feel like it. It helps to keep a flexible schedule. If you feel like sticking to it: fine. If you don't, DON'T! There are no generalities here. Everybody responds differently and has reduced energy but not depleted energy. I found books on tape very relaxing; they are available through our local library. Most insurance will allow for two wigs, it's fun to have a "funky" one along with one that looks like you. This is what my daughter did and enjoyed the "funky" one more. Your hair will come in curlier and stronger than it was so you have that to look forward to. Just take this on like a tiger by the tail. You have the best of the best in Dr. D. and she'll watch you like a hawk. Remember: NO QUESTION IS A STUPID QUESTION."

Laura (a 3 year breast cancer survivor and mother of two pre-teen daughters, diagnosed at first screening mammogram: 1. Have Benadryl & Senakot in your medicine cabinet. 2. Carry hand sanitizer with you at all times. 3. Plan to rest for a day or two after each chemo treatment. 4. Arrange for weekly Reiki treatments during the months of chemotherapy. 5. Don't be afraid to ask for help. 6. Talk to Dr. D. about a port so that IVs won't need to be started each week. 7. No manicures or pedicures due to risk of infection. 8. No hot tub. 9. The A/C combo (chemotherapy) is the worst. 10. Be kind to yourself.

TREATMENTS TO A CURE (CHEMOTHERAPY)

November 30, 2009

Dear Family & Friends,

Let me tell you about my day . . . I didn't sleep well of course in anticipation of this first chemo day. But even so, I went into the college today for my office hour. I had decided to invite the students to a Pre-Chemo Coffee Gathering. They had an exam this morning but still thirteen students showed up. Several others emailed that they had just missed me. I must share what our group of sixty students did for me. They bought me this great breast cancer scrub top and then they ALL signed it. Oh, and the students were very excited because they saw a rainbow on their way in to see me and believed it was a good sign . . . I agreed. I have shared this entire experience with them as I believe it will help them to be more caring, more hopeful, more positive, more knowledgeable and more prayerful when working with their patients one day.

They are on this journey with me and will always be a special group of students in my life.

So after the Pre-Chemo Coffee gathering, Brian and I made our way to Heywood Hospital to meet with Dr. D. and the chemo team. Dr. D. prefers no port as I will only have three more treatments with the really toxic Adriamycin/Cytoxan combination. I had no problem with it today. After the every other week of A/C, I will then have every other week of Taxol followed by six more weeks of radiation. At each treatment I receive my pre-meds for nausea and to prevent any reactions. Dr. D. is treating me very aggressively so that the CANCER never comes back . . . I am okay with that. So for several hours I sat in a lounge chair with Brian by my side in a room with patients being treated for all different cancers in all different stages. However, I must say that the love, hope, and support fostered by the oncology team was amazing. And I really enjoyed the visits from some friends too! Afterwards I actually had a bit of energy to visit friends in pharmacy, histology, maternity and Dr. C.'s group!

But now I am relaxing on the couch with my "nurse dogs" by my side just waiting for my side effects to hit me! Just kidding . . . actually I had a conversation with a good friend and I shared how relaxing, yet difficult, and stressful this will be because I am used to multi-tasking. She told me that I am multi-tasking . . . I am fighting cancer! You know, she's right! So my plan is to just keep being me . . . maybe those side effects are just what happens to other people!!!

Thank you for your love, support, prayers, emails, positive energy, etc . . . . please keep it coming. You are all fighting with me and it is making all the difference for me. Next chemo is December 14th . . . stay tuned!

Love,
Judy

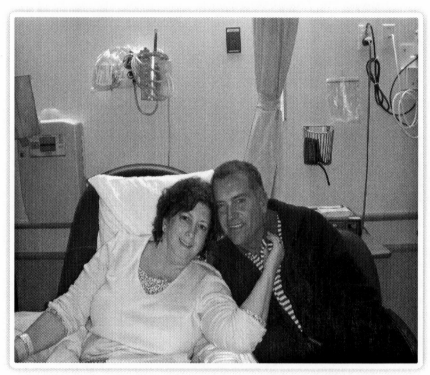

Brian and me at my first chemotherapy session

As I started my chemotherapy, friends and family wanted to help. So forever the teacher, I started to give out assignments. My best friend, Paula, was to make me my favorite pie dough dessert for every chemo session. Another friend, Vicki, was assigned to make me a batch of her special frosted cookies for my survival celebration (which she did the following July). And my friend Raeann did research on nutrition and cancer, recommending I eat Kefir (a natural yogurt type food filled with antioxidants for healing) daily. I did . . . all through my treatment. I can't eat it now without thinking of chemotherapy. Another friend, Meredeth, took it upon herself to organize a group of friends to make meals for the days when I was just too tired to cook. What a help that was! I was always used to being the one to help others . . . and as difficult as it was at times . . . I had to be okay with accepting help from others. Now as I reflect, I wonder what I would have ever done without them. I would pass that advice on to others living with cancer or any disease . . . allow others to help you!

* * *

December 5, 2009

Dear Family & Friends,

I was not going to send an update until after my next chemo date which will now be renamed "treatment to a cure," since chemo has such a negative sound to it. And we all know, and I often need reminding, that this is what the chemo is all about . . . to cure me of this breast cancer. I have decided to send an update now because it has been such a challenging week for me and your love and support makes such a difference.

Let me see . . . last time I wrote (11/30) I was feeling pretty good from the "Decadron" high . . . the steroid given to me with the chemo to make it more tolerable. On Tuesday, I even acused Dr. D. of giving me a placebo treatment. Well that lasted for two days before I "crashed" on Wednesday afternoon at which time I cried uncontrollably for an hour and a half. Finally I calmed down (with the help of some Ativan) but, the following day was just as bad. No vomiting, no nausea, no pain . . . . just incredible emotions. Some of you were recipients of my distress calls . . . please know how much having you listen and share kind words helped me. In the middle of all of this, Angel, one of our Italian Greyhounds . . . the one closest to me . . . had a seizure during the night Wednesday and again Thursday. My in-laws, Bob & Gloria, took her to the vet (thank you!) for us. Angel checked out okay except for a thyroid problem and some dental issues . . . but overall the vet believed that she was reacting to my illness. Our animal friends/family are so amazing! I think that next time I "melt down" I should share the Ativan with Angel!

Friday was a better day. Quiet and slow and relaxing . . . until the evening when we went to meet with the wig lady. Yes, I know it is only hair . . . and I have already prepared myself with the shorter haircut . . . but apparently my attachment is still there. I need to work on this because I will soon have no choice. Brian, Heather and Aimee went with me. And Heidi mailed me some interesting wigs from LA. But wigs are wigs . . . and not really me and certainly wouldn't look good on anyone with a red swollen face from crying! Monday evening, Heather and I will go to Look Good, Feel Good; a program offered by the American Cancer Society to teach women (and men) like me to use make-up, head wraps, wigs, etc. to feel better about how we look . . . very timely for me.

You know, I keep thinking of my research with Multiple Sclerosis in the PhD program. Those living with MS share the feeling that they must now learn to live with a "new normal" . . . this is what I must do also. I was sharing with some of my students the other day that I was worried that if the chemo is killing any "fast growing" cancer cells that might be hiding out . . . I am also worried that the chemo could possibly kill some of the "fast growing" cells that make me a better person. My students' assessment is that I may be experiencing anxiety and that my personality is safe through this process. When did the students become so knowledgeable??? They must have some good teachers!

Today is Saturday, I see snowflakes outside and I am actually enjoying watching them. Funny how our perspective changes as we pass through life's changes. Please know that I am okay . . . I am told that the next week will be better and will build me up for the 14th when we start all over again. Fortunately my schedule will become calm in the coming weeks. Thank you, thank you, thank you . . . how would I ever make it through this without all of you???

Love,
Judy

*   *   *

December 14, 2009

Dear Family & Friends,

Another treatment toward my cure today . . . and another bead added to my bracelet. Some of you don't know the bead story so I will share. I received a beautiful bracelet from some very special friends. I had been surfing the internet one day and discovered a site where they sell a collection of "empowerment beads" designed especially for breast cancer. At this site, 100% of the purchase is donated in memory of the owner's friend who died from breast cancer a few months ago . . . and there are no shipping fees. So I approached seven of you to see if you would be willing to purchase a bead for me to symbolize each treatment . . . I purchased the first for myself. So you see each bead will symbolize a treatment to a cure! For this week, a special thank you to Heather! I'm not yet sure how to "symbolize" the daily radiation for six weeks but I'll figure something out as the time approaches.

It's interesting to me in reflection that I have been feeling as if I am working as a private duty nurse. Please don't worry. I do have plenty of help. What I mean is that for my one patient (me) I have to be thinking all the time about what she needs and constantly assessing. Is she eating right? I know she doesn't like vegetables but I need to make sure she gets them. Did she take her vitamins today? Does she have a temperature? Is she protecting herself from infection? She can have an occasional drink but not too much, it's not good for her. Is she exercising? Is she napping? Don't let her get constipated (which is one of the side effects of the chemotherapy). Is she using her special toothpaste and mouth wash? Mouth sores can be another side effect. Did she take her Advil for the muscle aches? Is she sharing her feelings enough? Should I consult with another nurse? Or, do I need to call the doctor? And you know, she is not always the most compliant patient! There are a lot of things involved in caring for my "patient". And fortunately I have all of you to take care of keeping the positive energy and prayers flowing . . . so it looks like all of you are also on duty!

This past week has been a good one. I felt like myself, had energy . . . and my own hair too! My only "near melt down" was to find out a few days before I will likely lose my hair that insurance will not pay for my hair prosthesis (aka wig). I refuse, especially around the holidays, to pay any significant amount for one. Brian disagrees and thinks that it is an investment. I would rather donate the money to a better cause. Anyhow, I have a Santa's hat that will serve me just fine! And there are some very stylish wrapping paper choices out there! Actually, I do have the wigs that Heidi sent me and those of you who know Heidi know that she will make sure that I remain stylish through this whole journey! And there are "donor wigs" too which I am really okay with. So my friends please don't worry about my head . . . I've come a long way in a few weeks and am willing to cover it with just about anything. I was just upset with the insurance company . . . it seems like less and less is covered every day. Oh, I almost forgot, Heather and I went to the "Look Good, Feel Better" program last week and really had fun. There were three other women living through the breast cancer diagnosis. We were taught special makeup techniques and supplied with quality makeup donated by the cosmetic companies. Two of the women volunteering were breast cancer survivors and were amazing. So I tried some of the techniques on Thursday when I went to the hospital for my echocardiogram (one of the chemo drugs is toxic to the heart so I must be monitored). I went around visiting and received many compliments!

I'm realizing that I am a bit "chatty" this update . . . must be the Decadron! I feel that I am better prepared to manage the side effects this week or I'm hoping that I am. I have only a few obligations at the college this week but can otherwise rest up for next week when Santa comes! I have attached a picture of Heather and I today. I am journaling with photos and thought I would share this with you. The smile is sincere . . . not about the chemo but about being surrounded by people who care about me! My hair in the picture is mine but will likely be gone by Wednesday . . . it's now falling out at a rapid rate . . . ☺

Love,
Judy

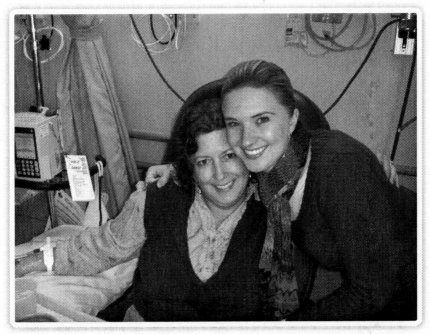

My daughter, Heather, and me at my second chemotherapy session

*   *   *

December 20, 2009

Dear Family & Friends,

I am almost half way through the "worst" of the chemotherapy . . . I am told that the 4 treatments of the A/C combination are the most toxic to my system. I can believe that this is true. This week has been better. Or I should say that I have managed it better. I now know that day 3 and 4 following the treatment are the "worst" days. So I was better prepared this time. I "lightened" my schedule, took my medications for nausea and relaxation, ate my veggies and my Kefir, and got plenty of rest. The physical symptoms seem to be managed okay but the fatigue is tough . . . I'm used to having much more energy especially around the holidays. Brian is doing a good job keeping energized enough for both of us! So I nap and rest as I need to . . . and I no longer feel guilty doing so which is an accomplishment for me . . . after all, I must remember that I am using the energy I have to fight cancer and to be healthy once again.

Oh, how could I forget . . . There was a traumatic event for me this week. My hair is now gone . . . temporarily. My hair was starting to fall out a hand full at a time so I made a decision after some consultation (thank you Nora and Chris, my brave breast cancer survivor friends). My sister-in-law Renee and brother-in-law Pat made a house call at my request on Monday evening. Renee buzzed my head with the love and care of a sister. I know it was a difficult thing for her to do and I hope she knows how much it is/was appreciated. I do have some wigs from Heidi . . . one in particular has received many compliments and one (the blonde) was a surprise for my students on their last day of the semester! And although I have never been a hat person that is changing very quickly . . .

So I sit now listening to Christmas carols, watching Christmas movies, admiring the Christmas tree and healing as we enter this holiday week. Without a doubt this is one of the most challenging times in my life but I cannot lose sight of all that I have to be grateful for . . . the cancer was caught early, the margins were clear, the nodes were negative, the chemo and radiation will kill *any cancer cells that might be hiding, my hair will grow back one day, my family will be together for the holidays, and I have the love and support of all of you on this journey. Thank you . . . I wish you all happy, healthy holidays! My next treatment is scheduled for the 28th . . . stay tuned.*

Love,
Judy

P.S. Angel is doing better but is still not 100%. She worries about me and is constantly "on duty" . . .

*　　*　　*

Losing my hair was so difficult. However it seems so insignificant to me now. I wrote the following in my journal not long after that evening . . .

More Things I Am Learning About Breast Cancer

That I am loved for me and not my hair . . . even though the nodes are negative and margins clear I still need chemotherapy . . . I need to buckle up and get ready for a bumpy ride . . . That there are others who have experienced chemo before me who will guide me through . . . That the internet is a scary place to learn about breast cancer . . . That there are people in this world way worse off than me . . . That I am not alone . . . That I am loved and supported . . . That chemotherapy begins again on Monday . . . That this is just some months out of my life . . . That my hair will one day grow back . . . That I must fight like a girl!

*　　*　　*

December 28, 2009

Dear Family & Friends,

December 28th . . . A/C 3rd treatment . . . another empowerment bead added to my bracelet (Thank you Heidi!) . . . one step closer to recovery. Tomorrow is my 50th birthday. I never thought I would be admitting this fact so freely. Imagine . . . this experience is actually helping me to view (or accept) some life events quite differently. Birthdays from this day forward will be a celebration of another year of life filled with love, family, friends, and life experiences. Birthdays will no longer be an event to dread. I've been telling some people that my theory is that the chemotherapy is killing the 50 year old cells and giving me 25 year old cells in return . . . See how I'm trying to remain optimistic!

The holidays have kept me very busy. Don't worry, I have still been resting frequently. I have really felt like "myself" this past week . . . well, all except for the hair situation. But even that is better. I will likely never again complain about having a "bad hair day"! After a few days of mourning, I have embraced my bald head (in private!) and have received many compliments on my new stylish wig. I have even experimented with other fancy head dressings. I have attached a family photo to demonstrate along with another photo of Heidi with me today for my treatment session. I tried to photoshop out the double chin but had no luck . . . I'm sure it was the photographer and not really me!

Our friends are here now from Germany. Actually they are more like family to us and I am enjoying their visit very much. It is healing for me. However, they understand that on Wednesday and Thursday I will need to be alone, likely with help from a dose of Ativan and/or Compazine and some comedy movies to help. From the last two treatments I recognize a pattern so I am now better equipped to deal with them. During those days when I need my alone time, Brian will travel with Henner, Marianne, and Andy to Boston, and to the Wrentham outlets. After those days, I will be able to enjoy more of their visit.

So once again I close with sincere gratitude to all of you. I have actually had many people tell me that I am one of the "best looking cancer patients they have seen". I accept this comment as a compliment and know that it is not a coincidence . . . it is truly because of all of your prayers and positive energy. And I freely share this fact. Please keep them coming and please accept my wish for all of us to have a happy, healthy new year!

Love,
Judy

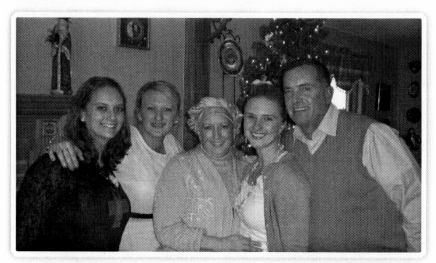

Our family at Christmas 2009, L>R Aimee, Heidi, me, Heather & Brian

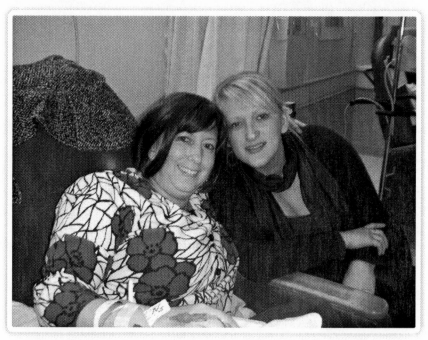

My oldest daughter, Heidi, and me at my third chemotherapy session.

*   *   *

January 11, 2010

Hello Family & Friends!

Yipppeee! The fourth (and last!) of the A/C combination and another bead added to my bracelet! Thank you to my sister Janice and niece Sarah! Still four more chemo sessions to go, but I am told they are with the "gentle" chemo. Do you really believe that there is such a thing??? But at least the worst seems to be over (I think and hope!) and I am one step closer to a cure! Although today I am feeling a bit worse than I usual do at this time. Must be the A/C build up in my body . . . oh well as long as it is doing it's job I will just have to handle it. I've been trying to strategically plan for the next round of chemo to coordinate with my teaching schedule. We return on 1/21 and I want to be "top of my game" on the days I am with my students!

Many of you were concerned when I didn't send an update last week. I actually thought that I was giving everyone a break from "Judy's Journey" only to discover that I worried many of you. I'm sorry. The week immediately following the chemo was challenging . . . even moreso than the others. Physical symptoms were controlled except for a few episodes of nausea. It was the fatigue that was so incredible. For every three hours awake I had to sleep for three hours! On New Year's Eve I took a nap in the afternoon, woke for supper, then I took another nap so I could "toast" in the New Year with Brian and my German family. Those of you who know me well, know that this is definitely not like me! This past week has been better though. I actually left the house and did a few things and felt more like my usual self. At least now when I pass through the "bad" days I do know that there are more "good" days coming my way! But there are days when I must "dig down deep" to remind myself about this fact.

I do have a funny story to share. I was doing a physical on a young boy this week while working for Dr. C. and the boy's mother told me that she loved my modern, stylish haircut. I thought to myself . . ." if she only knew" but I just smiled and said "thank you." What's even funnier is that I have been wearing a wig that Heidi once wore on Halloween as one of the three blind mice! She never thought that her mother would really need it one day! I'm much better than I was about the hair now and have adjusted. I still feel like myself with or without the hair. To be honest, there is part of me that is actually enjoying having no "bad hair" days! Don't get me wrong . . . I will still be happy when it grows back but I can wait until we make sure that the cancer won't grow back! In the meantime, I am actually finding myself enjoying the stylish wigs, hats and wraps. I have attached a photo again this update . . . my sister and me at today's treatment session.

Please know how much I appreciate your prayers, love, support, emails, visits, and cards. They are so motivational and inspirational. I am so fortunate to have the relationships I do with all of you. A wise mentor once told me that "it is all in the relationship" and once again he is right! Thank you to all of you *for being so special in my life. Next chemo session is scheduled for Wednesday January 27ᵗʰ . . . .*

Love,
Judy

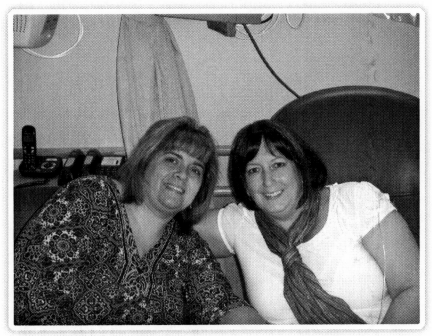

My sister, Janice, and me at my fourth chemotherapy session.

* * *

January 27, 2010

Dear Family & Friends

Treatment to a cure #5 today . . . and another empowerment bead added to my bracelet. Thank you Brian! Today was the new chemo drug Taxol . . . this is the one that is supposed to be "gentler" than the A/C combination. I certainly hope so but it does come with its own set of "adverse reactions". It was a six-hour treatment today complete with "premeds" for possible side effects and then the Taxol had to infuse slowly the first time. It makes me a bit anxious for the next few days to pass to see exactly how this will affect my body. I have strategically planned this treatment for a Wednesday . . . with the A/C combo my worst days were days 3 & 4 so if this remains true I can "crash" on the weekends. Thursday and Friday will be busy with two clinical days on Maternity surrounded by great students, supportive coworkers and happy moms and babies . . . all of which will provide me with positive energy! Oh, and I almost forgot . . . I started piano lessons this week. I've always wanted to and well . . . so I have some practice to do this week!

The researcher in me decided to try an experiment today. (See Dr. M., I may be on break but I'm still working on research!) I've been wearing my very stylish wig or my beautiful hat when out in public. When I wear these I receive many compliments and some people don't even know what's underneath. Today I decided to wear a head wrap. I happen to think the head wraps are also very stylish and draw attention to my strength . . . wouldn't you want the same? I've been worried that seeing me in a head wrap would upset others which would in turn upset me . . . this was my hypothesis. So today with Brian by my side for support I wore the wrap. Here are my findings: Mostly inconclusive. I have realized it is me that is more uncomfortable than the others. However, due to my small sample size and limited number of contacts today, I could not generalize my findings to the population of people seeing women with cancer wearing head wraps!!! A picture is attached for you to see for yourself!

Truthfully the last A/C combo was very tough. The symptoms which I was able to control with meds lasted much longer and the fatigue was even more incredible than before. During this time I actually thought I had a UTI (urinary tract infection). I wasn't sure and had read that the Cytoxen causes similar symptoms. So finally last Friday, when the symptoms became worse I was advised to come in for a urine sample. Turns out no UTI but I passed a kidney stone! Ouch!!! Apparently my poor body is so confused that it didn't have the traditional symptoms associated with kidney stones . . . or maybe I slept through them! But I have enjoyed five really, really good days since that episode.

Overall I continue to do extremely well and I continue to believe it is because of all of you! Thank you once again for your prayers, positive thoughts, hugs, emails, phone calls, cards, visits (it was nice to see you UP) and the beautiful flowers (thank you to the "church girls", Heather's special group of friends since childhood!). When I have "down" days, I reread the cards and emails and your words of support, love, and encouragement. Speaking of "down" days, in another email, I will share the "chicken coop story" . . . I think you will enjoy it. Hopefully I can sleep tonight . . . I think you can tell from the length of this that I am feeling the effects of the Decadron again!

Love,
Judy

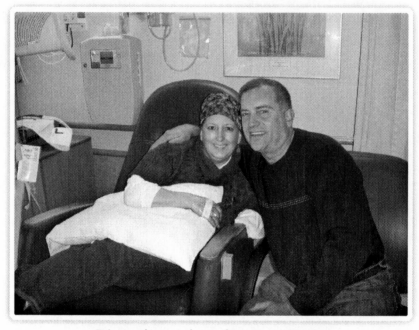

Brian and me at chemotherapy session #5.
I still can't believe he let me out looking like this!

*   *   *

February 10, 2010

Dear Family & Friends,

Treatment to a cure #6 . . . the 6th empowerment bead has been added to my bracelet. Thank you Renee and Pat! These empowerment beads symbolize each chemotherapy treatment. I wasn't sure how to symbolize the weeks of radiation but I think I have an idea. I am going to place a sterling "spacer bead" in between the empowerment beads . . . one to symbolize each week of radiation. My "cure bracelet" is looking very lovely these days, although I must admit it is getting a bit heavy with the weight of the beads . . . symbolizing the weight of my spirit some days and the inner strength needed. I must remind myself however that now I have only two treatments left. I have an appointment with the Radiation Oncologist for February 23rd and will learn more about the radiation plan at that time. Treatment to a cure #7 is scheduled for February 24th . . .

The "easy" chemo was not so "easy" on my body after Treatment #5. I ended up with a side effect experienced by approximately 60% of Taxol recipients. Beginning on the 3rd day post treatment I had excruciating bilateral leg pain from my hips to my toes. Fortunately, I had pain medication from surgery which I used along with some Motrin. Brian rubbed my legs with Absorbine Jr. at night and I slept in the spare room so that nothing would touch my legs. It was the worse pain I have ever felt in my life and lasted for four days. I have always been empathetic to my patients in pain but to experience it myself . . . well,

43

I had no idea of all that pain takes out of a person. My energy and spirit were "wilted" for a few days . . . but I have a plan this time. I will start Motrin on Thursday in hopes of keeping ahead of the pain as well as taking a stronger pain med for at night. Aunt Rosalie brought me some Biofreeze to replace the Absorbine Jr. My friend Margaret at MWCC gave me some reflexology exercises to try and my friends Kay and Diane have offered some Reiki if needed . . . . so hopefully this plan will work.

Bob & Gloria (Brian's parents) brought me today for my chemotherapy session. They were very impressed by the Oncology Unit at Heywood Hospital . . . and by the way the nurses care about each other and about their patients . . . and how careful they were with the medications and other tasks . . . and by how brave their daughter-in-law is! They really didn't say the last part, but I can tell they are proud of my strength and courage as I experience this challenge in my life. They join all of you in giving me the love, care, support, prayer and positive thoughts that keep me going. Thank you!

Life is otherwise okay . . . I have had to simplify my life a bit for now but am enjoying my family, my teaching schedule and my students, as well as some socializing during my "good days". I actually have about 4 or 5 before it is time for another treatment! I hope you are all doing well . . . please continue to keep me in your thoughts and prayers.

Love,
Judy

February 24, 2010

Dear Family and Friends,

Treatment to a Cure Week #7 . . . another empowerment bead added . . . finally a thank you to Aimee! Can you believe I have been at this now for almost three months . . . actually if we count the time from diagnosis it would be over four months! And you have all been on this journey with me . . . it seems like we may be reaching the half way point soon, when the chemotherapy ends and the radiation begins.

Yesterday Brian and I went to an appointment with the radiation oncologist, Dr. P. He was very knowledgeable and nice, but a bit concerned with the size of the bosom to receive the radiation. He actually asked if I still had a nursing bra around. I will admit that I can be a bit of a "pack rat" but after 23 years since the last time one was needed . . . off to JCPenney we went to buy a nursing bra. Good thing we explained to Heather first or she would have been wondering what we were up to when she met us at the store! Apparently I will need to wear a nursing bra during the radiation to keep the breast from moving or folding over and causing skin irritation or more radiation exposure than needed. I'm sorry . . . I'm sure the visual must be very scary for some of you! I also had to shop for all cotton, no underwire bras . . . and in my size they are very ugly but hopefully comfortable and supportive. Brian says they look like bras my Nana used to wear . . . so I'm wondering if I should be worried that he knows (or thinks he knows) what kind of bras my Nana used to wear!!! I have an appointment on 3/8 to prepare for radiation and then will start two weeks after the last chemotherapy treatment. I will require a total of 33 radiation sessions, five days each week until done. I plan to schedule for late afternoon whenever possible to avoid any interruption with teaching. Hopefully my plan will work.

The leg pain was slightly better with the help of some Percocet after the last treatment. However the Percocet made me very nauseous, so I was hesitant to take it. I have a new plan for this time around. I have a massage scheduled for Friday afternoon from a MWCC colleague. And will then take either a Compazine or Benadryl one hour prior to the Percocet to hopefully prevent the nausea which will ultimately take care of the leg pain at night and Motrin during the day. We'll see . . .

Oh, how could I forget! My most traumatic event since my last update was losing my eyebrows and eyelashes. I really thought I would keep them. I think this has bothered me even more than losing my hair. I have mastered the eyebrows with special makeup and "stencils". It's the eyelashes that are a challenge. The first morning I attempted to put them on, I called for Brian to help. Well he did try although eyelashes coming out of the middle of my eyelid might have not looked so natural! I really do wonder how many times I can drop the fake eyelashes in the sink and still have them be "clean"? Or how much eyelash glue I can get into my eyes without going blind? I actually have to get moving about a half hour earlier each morning to "put on my face, etc.". I feel like I am starting with a clean slate each time and could really look however I wish. However, I have realized that I am a much better nurse than cosmetologist!!! Heather is going to search for some "semi-permanent lashes" . . . certainly some must exist!

March 11th is the next (and last) treatment session, for chemotherapy. I still need all of you. Oh, and I have a special request for prayer/positive thoughts for my good friend, April, who was just diagnosed with brain cancer. It is inoperable, her symptoms came on suddenly and unexpectedly and at this time her prognosis is likely not as favorable as mine. I know how much your prayers/positive thoughts are helping me heal. I truly believe they could do the same for her. Thank you!

Love,
Judy

P.S. Looks like the Decadron is still in effect, even after being reduced this week! I have been chatty but there is a lot to share. I know many of you have shared my plight with your prayer groups, churches, and positive people in your life on my behalf. Please thank them and feel free to share my updates with anyone who is interested!

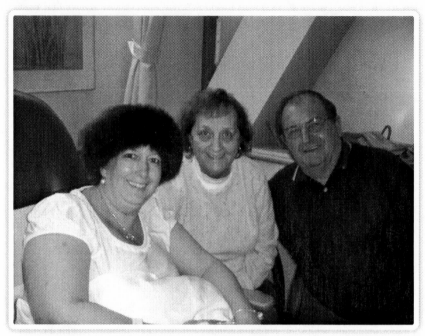

My parents-in-law, Gloria and Bob with me at chemotherapy session #6.
I am wearing my favorite hat!

*   *   *

March 11, 2010

Dear Family & Friends,

Yipppppppppppppeeeee! Yoooohoooo! The final chemotherapy session and the 8th bead added to my survivor bracelet . . . Thank you VBF Paula! Paula joined me this week to care for me and to celebrate the final session. My creative, caring best friend surprised me by celebrating with "gifts" of 8 . . . crazy 8s card game (that she actually thought we would play!), 8 of my favorite pie crust cinnamon rolls, 8 smidgeons (my favorite from Priscilla's Candy Shop), pasta shaped like survivor ribbons (I'm sure they are grouped in 8), the number 8 bead (not all went in order of the exact number), and a pink flower arrangement with a Breast Cancer ribbon on it (she tells me that the flowers are attached to 8 stems). My friend Diane stopped by with a beautiful bouquet of flowers also. Thank you! And the Oncology team gave me a cake with a certificate of completion and wishes for happy days ahead to take home. Thank you! The Pharmacology team sent over a card with a Godiva candy bar. Thank you! (Does anyone notice a common theme here? Something I must tackle soon). It was truly a celebration!

So to summarize to date: Phase I (diagnosis & surgery) was successful! ☺ Phase II (chemotherapy) was successful! ☺ And now we move on to Phase III: radiation. Heather joined me Monday to go for my radiation "simulation". That is the appointment where measurements are taken for radiation and teaching is done. It was very interesting. Well, that's one way to describe it. The decision made was not to use the nursing bra afterall. I think when I return it to the store I'm just going to say that I decided not to breastfeed . . . it will be much easier than the true explanation. So anyhow, if you can visualize this . . . . I will lay on my stomach with my left breast dangling down. The radiation will come from the sides to treat the breast tissue. It is a new technique used for larger breasts and will likely have additional benefits for me. For instance, it will be easier on my skin as there will be no skin folds treated and there will be less exposure to my lung tissue. My "tattoos" which are actually tiny dot markers are on my back and not my breast. The simulation had me in that position for 40 minutes! Fortunately the actual treatments will only last about 10-15 minutes. It's the travel back and forth X 33 times (daily except for weekends) and changing that will actually take most of the time. Oh well, at least there won't be chemicals running through my body!

These past weeks have been filled with many soulful thoughts. While watching the Olympics, we all learned of the beautiful young figure skater whose mother collapsed suddenly from a heart attack while watching the shows and two days before her daughter was to skate. This young woman made the decision to skate and performed exceptionally well in her mother's memory. There was a news reporter who wrote about the event/situation, his words remain with me now: "She was going to show the world the kind of woman her mother had raised by her decision to still perform." You know, I think this is also true for me. As I continue on this journey I hope I am also showing the world (and especially my daughters, family, students and friends) the courageous woman raised by two beautiful women (my mother and my Nana) who always encouraged me to be the best I could be. They are the women who taught me to be a good mother, a good friend, and instilled the importance of optimism, good relationships, and education in me . . . I'm sure they are smiling very proudly from heaven as they observe my challenging journey.

Please know I truly believe that I am doing so well because of all of YOU . . . I can feel the warmth of your care and support, your positivity and prayers and your love . . . Thank you!

Love,
Judy

P.S. Phase III emails to follow after first week 3/28-4/2 . . . I'll send an update then. Please don't worry!

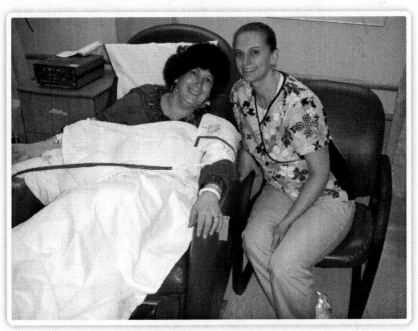

My youngest daughter, Aimee, with me at one of my last chemotherapy sessions. She was on her way to orientation at her new job as a registered nurse.

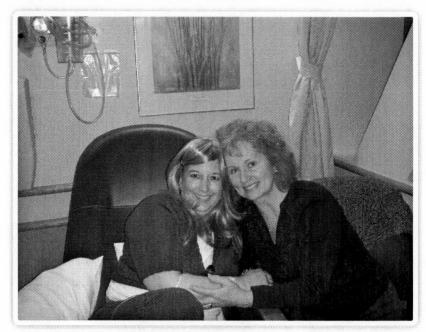

My very best friend, Paula, with me at my last chemotherapy session.
I surprised her by wearing my blonde wig!

*   *   *

RADIATION

April 2, 2010

Hello Family & Friends,

It's been several weeks now since my last update. I am doing very well, actually feeling more like myself now that my body is "chemical-free". Today was the end of my first week of radiation. A sterling "empowerment" spacer has been added to my survivor bracelet. Radiation is quite an adventure. In one of my past updates, I explained a bit about the process. But now that I have actually experienced it I will explain more . . .

My schedule is five days per week (no weekends or holidays), for a total of thirty-three sessions, not including the additional visits needed for xrays to confirm the area to be treated. I have scheduled my appointments for 4PM four days a week so that there is minimal interference with my work schedule. On Tuesday nights I stay at Heather and Corey's place in Lunenburg (about 2 miles from the center) and book Wednesday's

53

appointment early in the morning. This plan will save me a trip to Fitchburg as well as some fun to look forward to!

So I arrive to the Cancer Center at Burbank, check myself in by swiping my card, change into my johnny (hospital gown which opens in the front of course), put my valuables in a locker, put the locker key bracelet on my wrist, and sit in the waiting room to wait my turn. In just one week I have met some amazing people bravely traveling similar journeys. So it is my turn and I am escorted to the radiation room (the staff are very friendly), I lay flat on my stomach with my left breast dangling down and the right breast pulled around toward my back. I must lie perfectly still, which is not easy when there is "peppy" music playing . . . apparently I have more rhythm than I thought and moving my feet to the music throws off the landmarks. I notice now only classical music plays during my visits! So as I am lying there perfectly still this huge machine rotates around my body stopping twice to give the radiation. I can tell when it happens because of a loud sustained sound. The entire process takes about fifteen minutes. I have to take very good care of my skin because the radiation can burn it similar to a sunburn.

Good news during my appointment with Dr. D. (my medical oncologist), she doesn't need to see me now until August! However, she does expect me to lose 15 pounds by that appointment. If I can do what I have done in these past months, surely I can do this! I will plan to send an update each week as I pass through this phase of my recovery . . . unless I'm too tired, which I am told is a common reaction occurring more often as the weeks progress. Pictures will be limited as I go to the appointments alone . . . and based on the paragraph above, you can see that the pictures might not be appropriate to share! I'm sure the visual from my explanation is enough! I have attached a photo of me taken by Brian when we went on a Maine weekend two weeks ago. It was the weekend that the weather was sunny and in the 70s. We walked the Marginal Way three times. The first picture Brian attempted to take of us himself was a disaster. I didn't realize the wind had blown my wig so I had a 10 inch forehead and Brian's face was showing his curiosity about whether or not the picture would come out right!

I'm hoping that this update finds you all well. Spring is here and symbolic for me. Thank you for being by my side on this journey . . . I love you all!

Love,
Judy

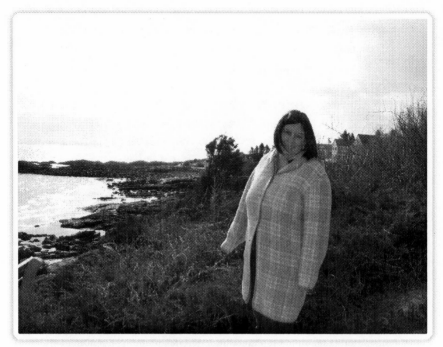

Here I am walking the Marginal Way in Maine. Brian and I had such a beautiful weekend!

*   *   *

April 17, 2010

Dear Family & Friends,

Fifteenofthirty-threeradiationtreatments done and another "empowerment" spacer added to my survivor bracelet! All is well so far . . . my skin is looking good, just a little pink but no blisters or pain. I will admit that I am tired at times but I'm really not sure if it is due to the radiation or just a busy schedule . . .

This week I realize how very lucky I really am. I know many of you told me one day I would see this journey as a blessing. This may now be evolving in my life. I know this from my new friends I have met in the radiation oncology waiting room. We see each other Monday through Friday as we wait for our turn at the radiation machine (there must be a special name for it but I don't know it). All I know is that the cancer center treats as many patients per day with one machine as their Worcester Center treats per day with three machines!

So we often wait and wait . . . and while we wait we share stories. There is Harry, who is my age, diagnosed eight months ago with Stage 4 lung cancer with metastasis to the brain. He never smoked a day in his life. His career has been to keep children safe and he is a jazz musician. He brought us all copies of a CD he recorded. The music is very relaxing and healing. He encourages me with my piano lessons . . . he thinks to master Jingle Bells is a great beginning for me! He often shares his embarrassment of losing his short-term memory. Most days he forgets my name but it really doesn't matter. And there is Molly who is also my age and a teacher, she is lucky like me . . . stage 1 breast cancer caught early on in a routine mammogram. She is even luckier because she still has her hair! And Hannah, who is also a nurse who is nearing retirement age. She had a lumpectomy that left her with lymphadema so bad that she can't close her right hand into a fist. Her daughter drives her to her appointments. She thinks that her working days are over. And Sam who just retired only to have his third bout with esophageal cancer and now must puree all of his food. And Scott who was diagnosed with anal cancer while going through a divorce. His physicians think the stress of the divorce contributed to his cancer. And there is Marlene who was just diagnosed with Stage 3 breast cancer and is having both chemotherapy and radiation together. She still works her factory job because she has to support her family. Every day I see the fear on her face. And Hilda, who is nearing 80 years old and has colon cancer which returned after just one year. She cried as she shared her story with me of marrying an American soldier and immigrating from Germany when times were so bad, only to feel that she is living in bad times here now in America. She has three children who live scattered around this country. She has not seen two of them in seven years. She calls me dear and encourages me by telling me how natural my wig looks and that my hair will grow back. It seems as though I meet someone new every few days . . . another someone on a similar challenging journey . . . another someone who still gives of themselves when they should be preserving this strength. Most of which are not as lucky as me . . .

So my dear family and friends, I think you will agree how lucky I truly am . . . and especially lucky to have all of you in my life praying for me and encouraging me. I am doing well now because of all of you . . . please share some of your prayers and positive thoughts with my new friends. I am feeling well enough to start to "pay forward" all that you have given to me. I will be forever grateful.

Love,
Judy

P.S. Names were changed to protect the privacy of those in the stories I have shared. No photo this week . . . no photo is needed . . . surely my words have "painted" a picture for you.

* * *

April 23, 2010

Dear Family & Friends,

Week four of radiation only had four days because of the holiday on Monday but still counts as week four in my book . . . the fourth spacer has been added to my survivor bracelet! And more great news . . . I am now able to climb the MWCC stairs to my office without feeling like I have to call 911! And . . . even more exciting is that I feel some eyelashes growing! Life is good!

Now, I realize that last week's update was quite "heavy" for some but the face of cancer is "heavy". It is real and is all around us, unfortunately it seems to be affecting more and more people every day. None of us are immune . . . I learned this first hand. However, how we deal with such a terrible diagnosis is what makes all the difference. It is the one thing we really can control. So in the radiation waiting room while we share our stories of sadness, we also share stories of hope, happiness and fun. And we laugh! We laugh at stories like the ones I'm going to share this week with you . . .

Months ago in the first week of chemotherapy, Dr. D. had dictated a note about my first visit. When I came in for the next appointment, Dr. D had flagged my chart to show me what had been transcribed. She had dictated "patient is in a PhD program and is preparing to start working on her *dissertation* soon." What had been transcribed was "patient is in a PhD program and is preparing to start working on her *disorientation* soon." !!! And, if anyone would have asked Brian all those months ago, he would have said that the transcribed statement was indeed the true one!

Last week, when changing in the radiation change room I looked in the mirror as I lifted off my top. I was shocked to see something dark under both arms. I thought to myself how crazy it was that my hair on my head was growing in light and now this . . . until I realized that it was lint from the new navy blue sweater that I was wearing!

Then this week, I went through the drive—through at the bank. I had my daughter's car which was low to the ground and not what I am used to since I drive a Jeep. I had trouble reaching the pneumatic canister to put in my deposit. As I reached further out the window to reach for it, my wig hit the top of the window and . . . yes, you guessed it . . . fortunately I caught it before it was all the way off but it was enough for the teller and the car in back of me to wonder what was going on. I just smiled (works every time!) and fixed it!

And then, there's the chicken coop story . . . I'll save that one for another time!

Wishing you all a week filled with love, good health and much happiness!

Love,
Judy

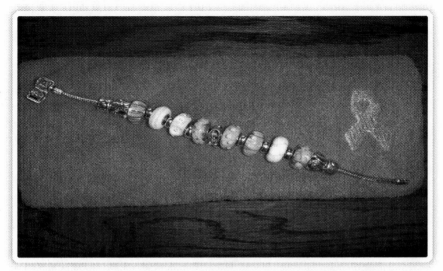

My Survival Bracelet. I always wear it to special occasions and times when I need strength.

*   *   *

May 1, 2010

Dear Family & Friends,

Almost to the end of treatment . . . 24 of 33 treatments done! My survivor bracelet is looking quite lovely . . . I will send a photo of it in a few weeks. All is well with me this week . . . a bit tired . . . the breast is a bit sore . . . I am a bit bored with my daily trip to the radiation center . . . but I am still smiling!

I'm hoping the radiation is affecting only my breast and not my brain. This week I came back from lunch break with my students after retrieving money from the ATM. The nurse's were a little concerned about me when I tried to security swipe myself into the nursery with my ATM card! And then one day, after taking a walk outside prior to my radiation session, I wiped my forehead due to the heat. On the spot where I wiped with my hospital gown, it was brown. I immediately started to panic, thinking that I had some type of side effect from the radiation. You can imagine my embarrassment when I realized that I had just wiped off my eyebrows! Oh, and my friend, Elaine, gave me a special blessing this week. More updates in next week's email . . . enjoy this beautiful sunshine!

Love,
Judy

*   *   *

May 8, 2010

Dear Family & Friends,

One more week to go . . . I thought this would be the last week but radiation treatment actually finishes up next Friday. I added the last spacer to my survivor bracelet but still have one more week. So I decided in memory/honor of my mother, my grandmothers, my mother-in-law, my heavenly mother, my sister, my VBF and all those who have "mothered" me through this difficult time in my life, I have ordered a "mother's love" bead (a heart with a pink zirconia) to finish off my survivor bracelet. You will all see it in the next update!

I had attempted to write and send this yesterday, and again this morning, but have realized I am just way too emotional. Finally, I decided to write this afternoon . . . afterall, I do always feel better when I share with all of you. I can remember one of you telling me this happened to you near the end. My breast has developed more radiation burns underneath which are painful. My doctor will not let me exercise, even walking, due to the "bounce" of the breast . . . apparently mine do it moreso than others. My hair is growing in ugly. Brian has been away on a much deserved vacation (which I could not go on due to radiation but encouraged him to go) . . . I miss him. Mother's Day's this weekend . . . I miss my mother. I miss Heidi. My class had their last day on Friday . . . I miss my students already. And I am just so tired . . .

So today I have given myself "permission" to rest! I cancelled any obligations that I had. I am sitting on my couch now, watching all my DVR'd shows. The rain is pelting against the windows and my "doggy" nurses are by my side. Believe me, they must be very glad I am getting better! I mean all of this "one-to-one" intense resting by my side over these months must be tiring them out! A few family members stopped by to visit, some friends have called to cheer me, and two very special friends (Thank you Nikki & Alissa! They are two young tween age girls who recently supported their own mother through breast cancer.) are coming tonight to make supper and watch New Moon with me. And best of all . . . I can feel myself healing!

Let me explain my thoughts for this week: The first is that of my students. It is after diagnosis but before treatment. They had all decided to give me a healing hug. There are many students who have supported me over these months. This is a very special group of students and I will always be grateful for their

*prayers and support. They will all be fine nurses!
The lessons learned this year are unique and
hopefully lessons which will enhance who they
are as people, and as nurses one day soon. My
special scrub top has been carefully put away
awaiting their pinning ceremony next year.
I wish them continued success in their second
year! The picture was taken about a year and
a half ago when visiting Heidi in California
with my sister-in-law and brother-in-law.
Brian and Pat were actually goofing around
with these wigs (I'm probably in trouble posting
this pic so please shhhhhhhhhhhhhhh!) . . .
little did any of us know that those two wigs
would become very important in my life!*

Love,
Judy

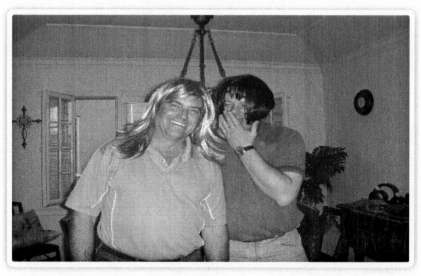

Brian and my brother-in-law, Pat, having fun with my wigs. I think they
look pretty good!

*   *   *

May 14, 2010

Dear Family & Friends,

Today was my last radiation treatment . . . 6100 rads total! *Today* I added my mother's love bead to my survivor bracelet! *Today* is the first day of the rest of my life cancer-free! In this update, I could focus on the grueling weeks of chemotherapy and all the side effects or the weeks of trips for radiation and the effects on my skin or the intense fatigue experienced at times or losing my hair and eyelashes and the hot flashes (both chemo-induced and hormonal) . . . but I choose not to. Today I want to share all that I have learned and continue to learn from this experience . . .

- I have learned to trust and believe in the divine power of prayer and positive energy. I have learned that we are not in control . . . God is!
- I have learned what really is most important in life. I have learned not to sweat the small stuff.
- I have learned that it really is true when you hear "something good often comes from something bad." I have learned to be open to the possibilities.
- I have learned not to save things until "later".
- I have learned that I am not loved for my hair, my eyebrows, or my eyelashes. I am loved just for being me! ☺
- I have learned that I have met new friends whom I would never have had

the opportunity to meet without this experience.

- I have learned <u>not</u> to trust the internet for medical information. It is just too scarey and often not very accurate!
- I have learned that pink is more than a color . . . it is a symbol of strength and survival.
- I have learned to smile more . . . is that possible??? ☺
- I have learned that all cotton, no underwire bras are actually quite comfortable.
- I have learned to like (I mean eat) spinach and asparagus.
- I have learned that only 10-20% of breast cancer patients have a family history and that the left breast is most common.
- I have learned to ask more questions.
- I have learned how important it is to share my experience to help others. If you know anyone who is newly diagnosed or struggling with the diagnosis of cancer . . . please give them my name. I want to pay forward for all the support I have received from others who have lived through this experience. I believe that I can help others.
- I have learned how to apply eyeliner.
- I have learned that I am resilient.
- I have learned that humor is powerful.
- I have learned how facebook works.
- I have learned I will continue to worry about the cancer returning. But I have also learned that worrying will <u>not</u> be

healthy for me. I have learned that I must be faithful with my follow-ups.

- *I have learned that today I must begin Phase IV of my recovery and lose some weight while increasing my physical activity. I have learned to be accountable to someone else for this will help me so when I send my monthly updates I will share my progress in this phase with all of you!*

- *I have learned that I must always be careful in the sun now especially in the area treated with radiation.*

- *I have learned that I enjoy journaling with pictures. What's that saying . . . a picture is worth a thousand words? How true! The pictures this week are: my own healing garden planted by Brian, and pictures of my radiation treatment. Oh, an update for you: When leaving church last week the Deacon commented to Brian about his photo. At that time Brian was not even aware that I had posted his photo . . . ooops!* ☺

- *I have learned I have raised three beautiful, successful, strong young women. Heidi, Heather and Aimee . . . you will always be my greatest accomplishment in life! I have been so amazed at your strength and ability to encourage and motivate me through this challenging journey. And, I must not forget Brian . . . I have learned he has come through for me in ways that I never thought possible. I love you all very much!*

- *I have recently learned that Brian and I are going to be grandparents . . .*

Aimee & Chris are due in January of 2011. I really like the saying that babies are God's way of saying that life should go on . . . how true! I will enjoy being a grandmother and am grateful to be alive to do so. Please don't worry girls . . . we still love our grandpuppies! ☺

- *I have learned without the love, support, and encouragement of my family, friends, and students (ALL OF YOU!* ☺*), I would never have made it through these past months. Thank you so much for being by my side!*
- *I have learned that I am a survivor!*

Love,
Judy

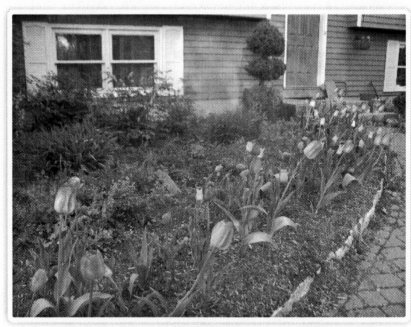

My Survival Garden planted for me by Brian.

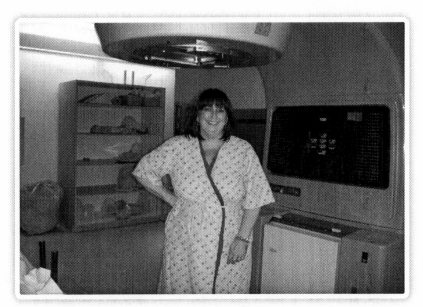

My last day of radiation.

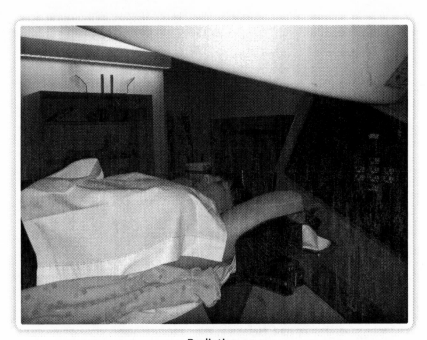

Radiation.

*   *   *

SURVIVAL!!! ☺

June 28, 2010

Dear Family & Friends,

How have you all been? I hope you are enjoying this beautiful weather. Please remember to enjoy all the moments . . . I have learned on this journey how important it is to do so. Today was my first follow-up with my radiation oncologist, Dr. P. All is well although he has encouraged me to lose 25 pounds before my next appointment with him in December. I think he is in "cahoots" with Dr. D. who wants this body 15 pounds lighter by the end of August. I know it is all in my best interest and imperative to live healthier in the second half of my life. And, as hard as it is to lose weight, I can't help but believe that after going through chemo and radiation I can do ANYTHING . . . including lose weight!

So I have "hired" my Heather to be my personal trainer. She is disciplined and extremely tough. Jillian Michaels is her idol, so if any of you have seen Jillian on Biggest

Loser then you know what I'm talking about!
I have been revving my fitness routine up . . .
Booty Ballet and climbing Runyon Canyon
when visiting Heidi in California ("before"
picture attached), walks with Brian around
the neighborhood and weights with Heather.
She tells me not to get too comfortable because
those activities were only "warm ups." My
plan is to share weight loss results with you
in future updates. ☺

Overall, I have been feeling really good . . .
great actually. I can feel myself getting
stronger every day. Others going through
this told me it would happen but when I felt
so badly I just could not imagine it. I will
admit that I do find myself trying to "catch
up" on all that I could not do while receiving
treatment. I have finally convinced myself to
"let go" and just focus on each day. Let me
share some of my days with you:

- I walked the survivor's lap at the cancer
  walk. It was very emotional, spiritual,
  and motivational. (picture attached)
- I "met" my grandchild. (picture
  attached)
- I shared my story with others newly
  diagnosed in hopes of "paying forward"
  for all the help I received from all of
  you. I look back through my updates
  and am just so grateful to be at this
  point. I could not see it, but all of you
  did. Thank you!
- Been visiting with old (and new)
  friends . . . and planning more visits.
- Went on a Girl's Weekend to visit Heidi
  in California with Renee, Heather and

Aimee. (*picture attached*). We had so much fun!

- I had my little bit of hair dyed. I was convinced it was the color (or lack of) that bothered me the more than the length. After three dye attempts the color finally took . . . only for me to realize that the length bothers me too. Oh, well it will grow, and in the meantime, I am grateful to have eyebrows, eyelashes, stylish wigs and beautiful hats!
- I did some extra teaching, physicals at HH and working some hours to help out Dr. C. All things that I enjoy doing.
- I am taking the time to smell the roses! ☺

My next update will be at the end of August. I wish you all a safe, fun and relaxing summer!

Love,
Judy

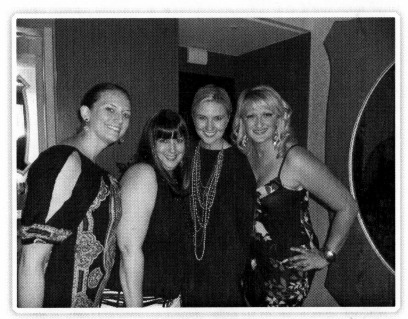

My first post-cancer girls weekend to visit Heidi. Renee is taking the photo.
We had so much fun!

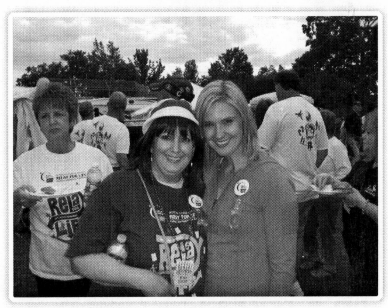

My first participation as a cancer survivor. My daughter, Heather, has
committed to walk this with me every year.

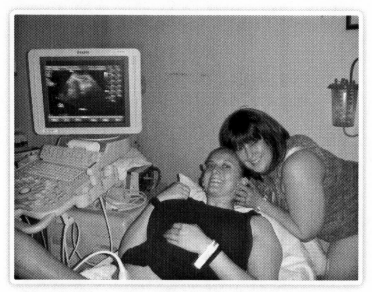

Aimee and me at her first ultrasound for my first granddaughter,
Jocelyn (on screen).

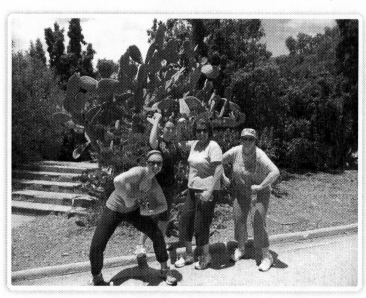

L>R Heather, Aimee, Renee and me. A very challenging climb up Runyon
Canyon in Los Angeles. This was a real struggle for me. Heidi walked
slowly with me . . . and helped dry my tears.

*　*　*

August 6, 2010

Hello Family & Friends!

I know some of you have been wondering how I've been doing, so I thought I would send you all a quick update. I am feeling GGGRRREEEAAATTT! :) I ditched the wig about a month ago and actually had my first "haircut" today. I didn't think it was really me, but today someone (another breast cancer survivor) asked who I was and that maybe this is the "new" me. She may have a good point. Since my last update, I have been exercising at least one hour a day six to seven times weekly. I am feeling stronger and healthier every day. Heather has been very strict but has made my fitness crusade fun too. I've kept busy with some "work" also . . . a bit of summer teaching and NP work for Dr. C. A wise friend once told me if you love what you do for work then it is never really work. I believe that is true in my life!

On Monday, Brian and I leave for our Germany/France trip organized by our friends, Marianne and Henner. The last time they saw me, if you recall, it was in late December during a chemo week. I was so sick . . . I'm sure they worried at that time it might be the last time they would see me. I will be always grateful to all of you for your prayers and support on this journey. I've actually been able to "payback" already by helping a few others which feels really good.

I have attached two photos, just of me . . . this email seems to be all about me! One is during our early morning (4.3 mile every morning) walk along the beach at OOB and the other is from today with my "first" haircut. I hope all is well with all of you. Please keep in touch. Next update will be at the end of the month after Dr. D's appointment . . . Take care.

Love,
Judy

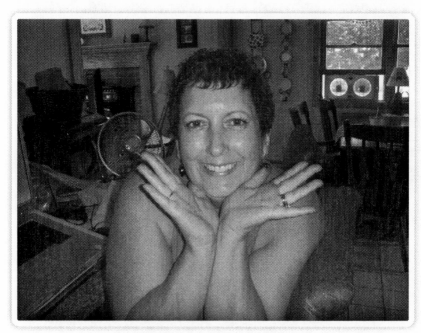

The wig is off! This was so liberating!

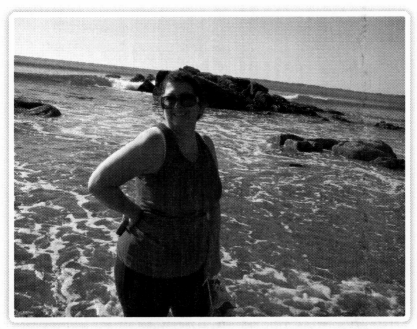

This is me on a fitness walk at Old Orchard Beach in Maine. By this time I really felt like I was gaining strength.

*   *   *

August 31, 2010

Dear Family & Friends,

Today was my first follow-up with Dr. D. All went well. She was pleased with my weight loss even though it was not the full 15 pounds that she had wanted me to lose. Heather, my personal trainer (aka daughter) wrote an "official" declaration of my summer workouts to "cover" me. Dr. D. said as long as the scale is going in the right direction she is happy. I had some lab work done and am just waiting for the results. She also ordered a bone density test for October and my first follow-up mammogram for November.

I remember one of my fellow survivors (I think it was Linda D.) warning me that now I might worry with each ache and pain that the cancer may have returned. Well, strangely for me, because I have been feeling so great I haven't been worried! I cannot imagine how this is possible, but rather than stress about it, I will just enjoy each moment and be thankful!

Our trip was fantastic! We had such a great time and I am so glad we went. Thank you Marianne and Henner for making it possible! I have attached two pictures from the trip. One of them is Brian and me in front of a well-known world landmark. The other is me with the French dessert I discovered called Profiteroles. Very yummy! (Shhhhhh, don't tell Heather or Dr. D!) The castle we stayed in was beautiful. Our room was in one of the back towers so I did get plenty of exercise walking up and down all the stairs!

We are now living in reality. My college commitments start tomorrow morning. Hopefully you have all been enjoying your summer. I'll be updating you all soon. Thank you for your continued love, support and encouragement . . . I am doing so well because of all of you!

Love,
Judy

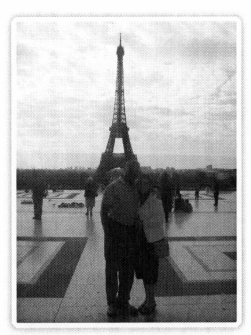

Brian and me at the Effiel Tower in Paris, France. We were on a wonderful vacation with our friends, Marianne and Henner.

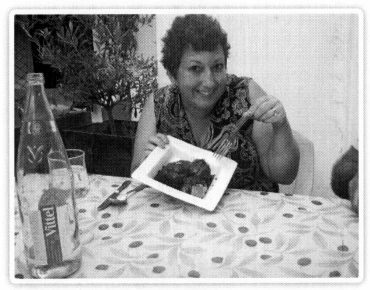

This is me in France eating one of my new very favorite desserts, Profiterioles. Yummy!

*   *   *

October 15, 2010

Dear Family & Friends,

This week marks the one year anniversary of my breast cancer diagnosis. It seems so long ago . . . almost like it never really happened . . . was this all just a dream? A nightmare? I was diagnosed on my daughter Heidi's birthday. So this year I took a trip to visit her . . . just a few days of mother-daughter time . . . to replace her "bad" memory with a good one. The other thing I did this fall was to participate in the local parade representing the nursing department for our college. I wore my special scrub top given to me by my students last year. I may have been representing the college, but in my mind I was celebrating my survival!

You know, I can remember last year when several of my survivor friends told me that one day I would marvel at all the good that comes from this experience. At that time, I couldn't imagine I would ever have those thoughts. I can honestly say I now understand. I feel different . . . I feel blessed . . . I feel grateful . . . I feel more alive than ever before. I seem to be more aware of the "little" moments than I ever was before the cancer.

I now truly understand what it means to "live in the moment". I thought I understood before . . . obviously I didn't. I was "rushing" through life, concentrating on my goals and not truly enjoying the moments of my journey. Thank you to a wise friend for helping me *to realize this. It took me a while and a life altering experience but I finally got it!*

So my plan for the second half of my life is to live healthier, enjoy the moments more, care more, love more, understand more, help more and stress less. At this point, I believe I am on track. Please continue to keep me in your thoughts and prayers especially on November 19th. My first post-treatment mammogram is scheduled on that day. Others tell me this landmark is one of the most emotionally difficult so some extra positive energy on that day will be most appreciated. I will be sure to update you at that time.

I hope this finds you all well and enjoying this beautiful fall!

Love,
Judy

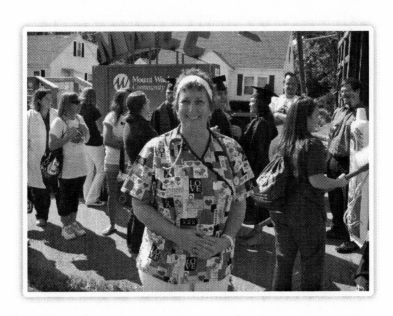

*   *   *

November 20, 2010

Dearest Family & Friends!

I am overwhelmed by your demonstration of love and support for me during this entire journey! And now I am so very grateful and pleased to share the good news . . . my 1ˢᵗ post-treatment mammogram is clear! Yipppeeee!

I must share this story with you. I lectured last week on Grief & Spirituality. I decided to share my story with this new class of students. There is just so much to learn from it. The students approached me after class requesting to start a new tradition of a "pre-mammo" tea. I met the class in the cafeteria this morning. So after "feeling the love" this morning, I drove to Fitchburg to meet a friend for brunch before my mammogram appointment. The traffic was slow due to route 2 construction . . . the license plate on the car in front of me said "LOVED" . . . I actually followed that car all the way to my destination!!!:)

I am doing well. Enjoying life. Living in the moment. Smelling the roses. Exercising. Eating better. Paying forward all the love and support I have received. Getting ready to become a Grammie. She'll be here soon and we are all ready. Aimee's shower was a few weeks ago and her room designed by Auntie Heather & Uncle Corey is done. I'll be sure to send my next update when she arrives!

Thank you! Danke! Merci! Gracias!

Love,
Judy

*   *   *

March 16, 2011

Dear Family & Friends,

Grammie told me that she really wanted to write an update to all of you so I asked her if I could help to write it this time. She has been so busy and happy since I came into her life. I have been too . . . I really have such a happy life with lots of people who really love me! But enough about me . . . let me update you about Grammie.

She's been busy with her teaching. She spends Tuesday evenings with me while Mommy and Daddy go on a date night and get a good night sleep. So when we have our time together, she tells me all about her life. She said that this semester teaching maternity is always her favorite. I think it's because she gets to play with other babies . . . probably because she misses me. And she said her students are really nice and they always like to see pictures of me!

Grammie has been feeling really good. She still needs to lose some weight and exercise more. I think I can help her with that because I really like to go for walks. She said a lot of people have been complaining about the cold, snowy weather this year but she really doesn't mind it much. She says I am her sunshine . . . in fact she sings that song to me all the time. She really doesn't have a good singing voice but it's okay . . . I love her anyhow and still like her to sing to me. She says she is really happy to be alive and that every day is a good day and she thanks all of you for always being there for her!

We hope you have a beautiful Spring!

Love,
Jocelyn XO

*   *   *

August 4, 2011

Dear Family & Friends,

How have you all been? I hope you are enjoying and cherishing life as much as I am these days. Each day I wake up breathing is a good day! I have intended to write an update earlier in the summer but I have been so busy . . . with good things though! Many of you have been encouraging me to publish my story . . . I have decided to do as you suggested. I spoke to a "self-publishing" company who seemed rather surprised that my purpose in publishing is to help others and not to make money! Today I have been reading through my updates in preparation . . . crying and laughing as I did so . . . much of my story I had actually forgotten . . . or perhaps repressed. Either way it is my survival story . . . and you are all very important characters in this story. The timing seems perfect for an update . . .

- *My follow-up appointment with Dr. D. in June went well. My second post-treatment mammogram was also negative. Future mammograms will be annually. She only has one concern now . . . yes, you guessed it . . . my weight! A common theme for many of us. It took all my energy to battle cancer last year so now I must use all my renewed energy for the battle of the bulge! Wish me luck! ☺*
- *My girls are great and keeping me very busy! Heidi and Ainsley are having a baby girl, Ivy Rose, in November 2011.*

Heather and Corey are engaged now and having a destination wedding in April 2012 followed by a Mr. & Mrs. Celebration in June 2012. And Aimee & Chris are making Jocelyn a big sister in February followed by their wedding in May 2012. So as you can see Brian and I are very, very busy these days!

- Tuesday evenings are still reserved for Jocelyn! She is a happy baby and has brought so much joy to all of our lives! I look forward to welcoming her sibling and cousin soon! When we spend time together there are no worries . . .

- My class of students . . . whom I shared with at the beginning of my journey . . . graduated in May. I was asked to be the speaker at their pinning ceremony. I was so honored to do so and very proud of each and every one of them. I have attached a copy of the speech in case any of you might be interested.

- I walked at the Relay for Life walk again this year . . . . with my own hair (four haircuts already!) and another year of survival to brag about! Thank you to all who donate in some way to this important event!

- I continue to meet with my special group of colleagues who have been affected by cancer. We continue to have new members. I hope to see the day when these types of support groups are not needed. That we meet just to enjoy each other's company. When cancer is only read about in the history books . . .

Next update will likely be around the holidays. But please know that I am here for you or others that you may know . . . who might benefit from my story of survival! In the meanwhile, I wish you all sunny days and warm hearts and positive energy and many, many beautiful moments.

My love to all,
Judy

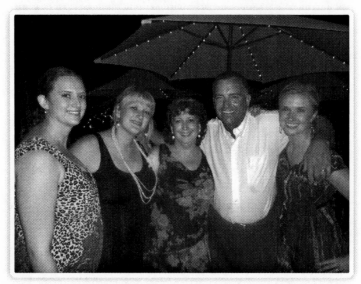

Our family celebrating together at my nephew's wedding. L>R: Aimee, Heidi, me, Brian and Heather. We had so much fun together. And the family will always remember our stay at King's Inn!

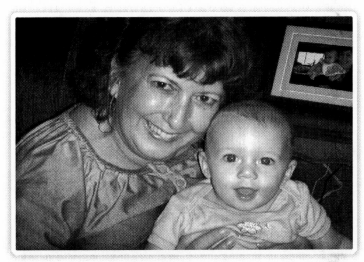

Here I am with my first granddaughter, Jocelyn, on one of our Tuesday nights together. I thank God everyday for giving me more life to enjoy this . . . and two more granddaughters, Ivy and Zariah, were born later in the year!

* * *

September 24, 2011

Dear Family & Friends,

As we approach my two year anniversary (October 15th) of surviving breast cancer, I thought I would send you a quick update. This week I have had to make an incredibly difficult decision in my education plans. As most of you are aware, prior to my diagnosis I had been pursuing my PhD in nursing. Actually I had traveled quite a distance in that journey before life gave me a detour. I must admit with that detour came another journey complete with new goals and dreams.

My oncology team has confirmed my concerns that the additional stress on my mind, body and spirit of continuing to pursue my PhD would not be in my best interest. I am a bit disappointed, but know in my heart this is true. By choosing to not continue toward this education goal, I am feeling I have left something that was important to me unfinished. However, there are many other things in my life now which are also important to me. I have been blessed with more time in life and I need to use it wisely. I love my job as a nursing professor at the college and my plan has always been to continue to work in this role. My original purpose in pursuing the PhD was to be a better teacher. Believe me when I say I have learned so much in the program. But I have also learned so much from journeying through cancer. And because of both experiences I truly believe that I am a better person and teacher. Perhaps sharing my story and helping others, as well as participating in the lives of my grandchildren, are areas where I will make my greatest contribution in life. Being so close to death certainly changes one's perceptions on life.

I have started to work on my book but had to take a break from it. Reliving that year in my life is very emotional. I am reading entries I don't even remember writing. I was in more emotional, spiritual and physical pain than I had realized. In some pictures I actually looked sick . . . at the time I thought I looked good. When I asked Brian how he could let me go out looking so sick, his reply was he didn't see it that way . . . he was just happy I was breathing, alive and able to go out. This is likely how many of you thought and I thank you from the bottom of my heart for your encouragement and inspiration.

Next month I am planning to walk toward a breast cancer cure with a fellow survivor. Her name is Wendy and at age 36, beautiful, smart, athletic, married with two young daughters, was diagnosed with breast cancer. Her breast cancer was more advanced than mine requiring her to have a double mastectomy, chemotherapy, radiation and multiple corrective surgeries with another scheduled in November. When she was first diagnosed, I shared my story with her in the hopes of paying forward the encouragement and inspiration that had been shared with me. It was interesting that she was also diagnosed in October. I promised her at that time I would walk a survivor walk with her. The good news is she is doing wonderfully and has reminded me of my promise to join her in this cause. It is not a 60 mile walk, only 3 miles, but just as important. I will send information in a separate email. Please consider donating in my honor and that of every woman . . . even $1 makes a difference! Thank you!

Love,
Judy

*   *   *

I was not able to participate in the Breast Cancer Walk as I had intended. It was a promise I had made to my friend Wendy. However, Brian agreed to walk in my place. He was amazed at all the people who were affected in one way or another by breast cancer. I worried about him while I was going through my journey. Was he okay? Who did he have to talk to about it? I believe this event helped him in so many ways. He has often shared how this event gave him time to reflect and helped to give him a sense of closure.

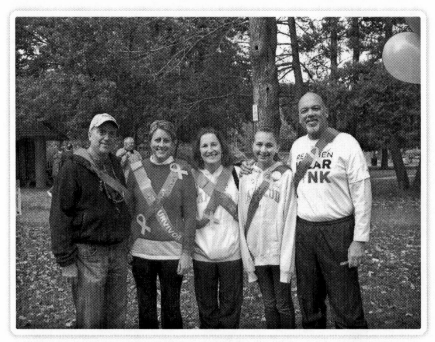

Brian (the only one wearing his sash backwards) at the cancer walk with our friends, Wendy (fellow survivor), Shelly (fellow survivor) and Shelly's daughter and husband. I was sorry to miss this walk. Brian had said that it was a life altering experience for him.

As I was preparing this manuscript, I realized how important it is to share the thoughts of those individuals who were important to my recovery. Of course there were many others whose prayers and encouragement helped me along the way. They know who they are and how much I will always appreciate them being there for me. However these were the individuals in my immediate circle. I did not realize how difficult a request I made when asking them to share their thoughts. Remembering is difficult for everyone, not just the person with cancer. It might be similar to asking a soldier to describe their role in fighting a war. A few of my "soldiers" were willing, or should I say able, to share. Others were not ready to do so.

Brian (my husband):

"When Judy first told me that something was suspicious on her mammogram, I didn't know what to think. So I just figured I wouldn't think about it until the actual reading by the doctors. When the results were positive, I realized how little I knew about Breast Cancer. I also knew that I was about to learn much more on the subject. I knew it was my responsibility to go with Judy to her appointments and listen intently to the plans for her treatment.

I viewed our situation to be an obstacle which we would overcome together. There were only two occasions when I briefly began to think of worst case scenarios. I worked hard to avoid that type of thinking. I really didn't feel it would be helpful to either one of us. My goal was to stay positive at all times. It gave me strength to know she was getting the best possible care and that all the positive energy around her would help us in so many ways."

Heidi (eldest daughter):

"When I found out about the diagnosis it was very difficult. I was 3,000 miles away and felt helpless. I didn't have the support group of the rest of my family and also felt a huge obligation to seem strong when speaking with my mom and my family back east. There were times I would cry in my room and imagine moving back, getting married having children all as soon as possible in order for my mom to see these important life changes. It was a very sad and trying time. I had no one to talk to about how i felt and my friends were afraid to mention it at all which I took for them not caring. When a diagnosis like this happens you are in a fog. Suddenly nothing in my life seemed important anymore. Daily activities such as work became robotic since my mind was focused on what my life would possibly be like without her. It was an unimaginable feat. There was also guilt for moving so far away and losing out on precious time. You never think of your parents possibly dying. Not at their early 50s and I had fear I wouldn't be able to handle it. Through every part of the process we began to get a glimmer of hope that she would beat it. Her positive attitude is really what kept me together. There's nothing that prepares you for a diagnosis like this. I never imagined my seemingly healthy young mom getting sick. Thank God she beat it! We need her around as there are so many more memories to make. Love you mom!"

Heather (middle daughter):

"First hearing the words from my mother, "I have breast cancer," sent chilling and frightening thoughts through my mind. For as long as I can remember, I have always connected the word "Cancer" with "the end". So naturally I was devastated to hear this news. My mom is my best friend and I could not imagine my life without her.

My mother has always been an inspiration to me. The way she is always thinking of others . . . her strong work ethic and value of education . . . the fun she has with those she loves. Wherever I go, there is always someone telling me how wonderful my mother is and how fortunate I am to have her in my life. I always smile and say, "Thank you. I know". I just knew in my heart that my mother had so much left to give in this life and that cancer could not take her from all of those that love and appreciate all that she does each and every day.

When my mother was first diagnosed, I could tell that she was scared. While some people may let fear consume them and run their lives from that point on, my mom turned to positive thinking. After the initial couple days of shock, she began fighting the battle with a smile on her face and an optimistic view for the future. She began writing about her experience in living with breast cancer and sharing her journey with others. Her writing was filled with positive insights and lighthearted stories about her journey. This writing proved to be very therapeutic . . . not only for my mother, but for those reading it.

Each and every day, I continued to be amazed by the way my mother took something so negative and turned it into something so positive. I kept thinking to myself, "How is she doing it? How is she continuing to be everything to everybody while facing this?". Every step of her journey living with breast cancer proved how resilient my mother truly is. My mother is an amazing woman, for all that she has done in her life and for all the lives she has touched over the years. But most of all, she is an amazing woman for the way that she continues to positively influence others as she shares her powerful journey living with breast cancer and overcoming fear.

My mother's journey has impacted my life in so many remarkable ways. I find myself living more in the moment and stepping back to take a look at the bigger picture in life. I find myself sharing positive thoughts and words with those feeling down and troubled by the weight of their personal situations. I find myself not afraid of all that I once was afraid of. More than anything, though, I find myself smiling, knowing that my mother, my best friend, will be around to share in the love, laughs, and memories that have yet to come in our lives!"

Aimee (youngest daughter):

"When I finished nursing school my parents had asked if I would be their HealthCare Proxy. I agreed and planned to take my honored role very seriously. However, I had no intention of my mother needing me to make health decisions for her yet. I did feel the need to discuss it with her though just in case. In my heart, I knew she would be fine. She always is. She is a very strong woman. She is the "go to" person in our family. I was the first daughter she told of her diagnosis. I think it was because I am the other nurse in the family and she thought I would understand. I did but I still wished that it was not affecting my mother.

One of my funniest memories was when I came home from working the second shift. It was midnight and my mom had left a note on the refrigerator. It said "Pizza in fridge. Bald mom in bedroom." It was the night my aunt had shaved her head. At the time, it gave me comfort to know that she still had her sense of humor. I kept that note on my own fridge until just recently. It still makes me laugh when I think about it."

Janice (sister):

"Judy and I have gone through a lot of heartache over the past 20 or 30 years. We lost our wonderful mother, Grandmother, Uncle and other loved ones who rocked our world. We had mutual experiences with children going through tough times as they were growing up. Through these times we had each other. We could talk and comfort each other. We could support each other because we both had experienced the same trials. We shared our faith and dreams for our families and watched each other move through the dark times and onto new beginnings.

Then one day Judy told me that she had breast cancer. I didn't know what to say. I didn't know what to do. The sister that I loved and counted on to be there always was faced with a serious health condition that could possibly take her life! This was an experience that I had not gone through before and the person I looked to for answers was in the middle of this crisis. I knew that I had to be there for whatever Judy needed. I would have done anything to keep Judy from going through this trial but I couldn't. I didn't know how to support her but I knew that God would show me how to be there for my sister. Judy was so brave. She never complained. She developed a spiritual strength that I had never seen before. Her body may have been going through the worst physical trauma it had ever experienced but her mind and spirit grew stronger and stronger each day. I am proud to call Judy my sister! Love you sis!"

Gloria & Bob (parents-in-law):

"When we first heard of Judy's breast cancer we thought the worst. As time went on we had more positive thoughts that everything would turn out good. She had such a large support group during her chemotherapy and radiation treatments. We were happy to be able to support her by sitting with her during one of her chemotherapy treatments, as well as helping in any other way she needed us. She is now on the road to being her "old" self and everything looks very good for her to live a long life."

Paula (best friend):

"How do you put into words or say the right thing to your very best friend who you love so dearly, when she asks you to give her the results of her breast biopsy while you are at work. The day had approached the final results of her breast biopsy were in. I was praying to "God" please let the results be negative as I was looking them up. The results were positive. It was as if all my blood had just rushed out of me as my very best friend was waiting on the phone for her test results. I called, upon "God" to give me strength and courage as I gave my very best friend the worst results anyone would ever want to hear. The conversation was strange, I could feel the love and sadness we were sharing. She thanked me and all I could say was I am so sorry. As I hung up the phone, I was crying uncontrollably and asking "God" WHY!!!!!! This was one of the worst things I have ever done in my life. While I was thanking God for being with me, I was also questioning Him, WHY? . . . . I did not like or understand His plan. "God" always has a plan and a lesson to be learned by all as we travel life's journey . . . I prayed like I had never prayed before, I was praying for healing, comfort, protection and love. I prayed throughout the day until I was able to leave work. I went immediately to Judy to give her a hug and tell her I loved her and that I would be there for her."

Bernadette (former nursing student):

"I clearly remember the day our dear instructor, Judy, shared with us her diagnosis of breast cancer. A small group of classmates and I were in our first clinical setting, we were nervous and unsure of ourselves. Judy guided us with her encouragement and reassured us with her gentle, calm presence. Even in the telling of her new burden, her strength was remarkable, but she allowed us to see enough of her vulnerability to share a round of hugs."

In the weeks to come, she maintained professional composure and moved forward with determination and grace, always willing to teach us about procedure, medication, and side effects related to her ongoing treatment. Her humor allowed us to laugh with her when wigs became a new part of her wardrobe, and in her playful way modeled a Pocohontas wig for added fun. Judy always looked super cute and never looked sick. It never, not once, occured to me that this disease could beat her. She is the very essence of healing and strength. Although she readily surrendered to the process of diagnosis and treatment, she never surrendered to the disease."

END NOTE

My story does not end here. My story continues. There will be ups and downs I'm sure. I am also sure my faith and optimism will be challenged but will ultimately enhance my survival. I will be forever grateful for every extra moment of life that I am blessed with. Every day I wake up is a good day. I find joy where I often failed to look. I struggled in the beginning, when first diagnosed, whether or not to share with others. For me, sharing made all the difference in my survival. Please don't be afraid to share or to encourage others in similar situations to do the same.

I would encourage you to remove all negativity from your life or from that of your loved one. Living with cancer is like fighting a war and happiness is one of the few things you can control. Only positive thoughts and love can be allowed during the healing process and into survival.

Another very special thing I have done for myself is to join a support group. Not all support groups are the same. You must fine one that works for you. We are a group of health care professionals who are now cancer survivors. We call ourselves the *Cancer Travelers Extroordinaire.* We meet every other month and share our fears and hopes, love and laughter. We share in a way that only fellow survivors can.

A wise friend advised me that there are times when we are detoured on our "path" in life, when our scripted story changes on us and we feel that we have lost control. Those are the perfect times to reflect on our lives; past, present, and future and to open our hearts and minds to scripting a new story . . . with our own new happy ending. I think that he may be right . . . he often is . . . and he enjoys being right.

Whether you are newly diagnosed with cancer, journeying through treatment or just interested in the subject, I am hopeful that you have gained some insight from my story. It is unfortunate that cancer still exists in our world. We need to comfort, support, and encourage one another. We need to share our stories and learn from one another. We need to continue to believe in a cure one day.

ADDENDUM One:

Pinning Speech given to nursing class of 2011 on May 20, 2011:

President A., Dean C., Director C., Esteemed colleagues, Honored Guests and most importantly the graduating nursing class of 2011 . . .

Let me begin with congratulating our nursing class of 2011! For those of you who have not met me, my name is Judy Fredette and I am a nursing professor, teaching freshman nursing. I teach fundamentals and maternity. However, I don't believe that this is why I have been asked to speak to the graduates today. I believe that it is because of my role as a survivor. While I have been journeying through and surviving Breast Cancer, this group of graduates has been journeying through nursing school with their own individual survivor stories! I'm sure that our survivor stories overlap and intertwine in many areas. For me, many of these graduates have played an important role in my survival. But today is not about my story . . . today is about theirs . . . today is about the nursing graduates who sit before you . . .

Please know how very privileged and honored I am to be asked to share my thoughts with you today. I have much to say, I usually do but with limited time to say it all . . . especially with 108 nursing graduates receiving their nursing pins tonight. Because of this I have decided to share in a manner in which our nursing students are taught . . . clear, concise and accurate . . . and I will use the nursing process as my foundation for these thoughts! For those of you non-nurses, some of what I will say may sound like a foreign language. For the graduates it will make perfect sense.

*Let me begin with my **assessment** . . . My assessment, and I am sure that my colleagues would agree, is that before you sits a group of caring, well-educated, well-prepared, and clinically safe new nurses. To adequately complete and focus my assessment I will use Gordon's functional health patterns which are well known to all of our students.*

Health Perception-Management Pattern: *The students have learned to multi-task in a variety of roles . . . mothers, wives, sisters, daughters, husbands, fathers, sons, nurse aides, and friends as they have done this. Some have been able to keep balanced while others have leaned in one direction or another as a matter of temporary survival.*

Nutrition-metabolic Pattern: *This pattern has varied among the students. Some have continued to eat healthy, some have started to eat healthy and others have been seen to have maintained on twinkies and soda. However, the specifics are confidential.*

*We'll skip over the **Elimination Pattern** . . . and move on to . . .*

Activity-Exercise Pattern: *Another functional health pattern in which the findings are varied. Some have maintained exercise, some have started exercise and for some the only exercise they have had time for is to turn the pages of their textbooks!*

Sleep-rest Pattern: *This is also a pattern with varied findings dependent on a variety of factors. Were the* students in the evening or day or bridge program? Were they working? Did they have family obligations?

Cognitive-Perceptual Pattern: Generally one would assess pain level on a scale of 0-10 . . . . some students may have found the nursing program to be more "painful" at a 10 while others would describe it as less painful on this numerical scale. I believe that Graduation and passing NCLEX will surely take care of any of this pain!

Self-Perception-Self-Concept Pattern: Although I have not had the opportunity to get to know each student personally, my assessment would be that to arrive at this point in their educational career . . . every student must have grown significantly in their self-perception-self-concept . . . and they will continue to do so as they journey along in their nursing career!

Role-Relationship Pattern: This is the pattern where all of our honored guests deserve credit. Many of you have made all the difference in "making it work" for your particular nursing graduate. They are sitting here because of all of you. Very often sacrifices were made for this to become a reality. Your patience, support and encouragement will always be remembered by this group of graduates!

Coping-Stress Tolerance Pattern: The fact that this fine group of graduates sits before you smiling is the best observation for the assessment in this functional health pattern!

Value-Belief Pattern: The students have surely evaluated and re-evaluated this pattern themselves throughout the program. One value-belief that I am sure that they all share is the belief that they would one day sit here before you.

My assessment is now complete . . . Next I must make my nursing diagnosis. There are many nursing diagnoses from which I could choose but today I choose : Fear r/t NClEX exam aeb students expressing fear of taking this certification exam.

Some recommended interventions are:

- Believe in yourself as we believe in every single one of you!
- Study . . . . study . . . study!
- Critically thinking . . . for this exam and forever!
- Use your ABCs . . . . airway, breathing, circulation!
- Your first answer is usually the correct answer!
- Take deep breaths!
- Celebrate your success!

The rationales for these interventions should be very obvious to all of our students. We have prepared you well. And our realistic, measureable, time framed goal is that: Our students will express a significant decrease in fear after passing the NYCLEX exam! ☺

So you see dear graduates, "Life is a Care Plan" . . . we are continuously assessing, re-assessing and prioritzing our goals, dreams and accomplishments. We diagnose our situations along life's journey, devise our interventions all the while considering our rationales to reach our measurable, realistic, time-framed goal. As life goes on we re-evaluate this "care plan" and the process begins again.

In closing, I want to share a quote that I often share with students and colleagues: "Just as children are a direct reflection of their parents, students are a direct reflection of their teachers". Please continue to smile, think positive, and be kind! We are all very proud of you! Let's give our nursing graduates and all of us who contributed in some way to their success a BIG HAND! Congratulations!!!

ADDENDUM Two:

The Chicken Coop Story

It was the third day after my first chemotherapy session, a Wednesday. I wasn't prepared for this day. Monday and Tuesday had been challenging but in a much different way. I was surrounded by supportive family and friends. This was the day when everyone thought I would be okay. And so didn't I. I was sadly mistaken.

Brian had gone back to work. I was home alone except for my "nurse" dogs, Daisy and Angel. They were doing their best to support me. My physical symptoms were bad . . . nausea and vomiting, general malaise, headache . . . but my emotional symptoms were much worse. Reality hit me hard. "I am dying . . . this is it . . . I know it." These were the thoughts going through my mind. I began to cry uncontrollably. After about an hour in this state, I had what I thought was one of my first rational thoughts . . . ." Brian has always wanted chickens. And I have always said NO! So if I am now dying then I should at least make Brian's dream come true and do it in time to watch him enjoy it."

I remembered how while taking a joy-ride a few months prior that Brian had admired a chicken coop he had seen for sale. It was a beauty as I recalled. Complete with comfy "apartments" and it's own "heating system". Those would be very happy chickens which would make Brian very happy. And when he didn't have me around, the chickens would be comforting to him. I was sure that this was a plan worth pursuing. So in the midst of my tears I called the store where we had seen the chicken coop. The salesperson told me how there had been a lot of interest in this very special chicken coop and that it was selling for $2000. After more discussion, I hung up very pleased with myself that I had talked him down to $1700. But that price was only good for the next few hours and with delivery the following day. After a few moments, I realized that I had no idea where I would get $1700, especially a few weeks before Christmas. So the tears returned full force.

Suddenly it became very clear to me. I would call my daughters to see if they could "chip in" towards this chicken coop. Time was ticking away . . . I had only hours to make Brian's dream come true before I died. I decided to call Heidi first. It was about 3PM EST so she should be at lunch now in California. I reached her right away and excitedly shared my plan and asked for her help. "You are going to do what?!" was her response. I hung up quickly after some "small talk" realizing that Heidi would not be the one to help this dream come true. "Okay" I thought to myself. "She just doesn't understand. If anyone is going to help me, it is Heather. I'll call her next. Surely she will understand."

Knowing that Heather would have just finished her teaching day, I called her. Again, I excitedly explained my plan. "Mom, do you know how many eggs Daddy can buy with $1700!" was her reply. Again, I made some small talk and hung up. How terrible that I would not be able to make Brian's dream come true before I died. I didn't even bother calling Aimee, the practical one. If I had convinced Heidi or Heather, I may have had some luck with Aimee. But I knew that it was useless now. And honestly I couldn't take any more disappointment. So I cried and cried and cried. Finally in desperation, I called the oncology unit where I was receiving treatment. Through my tears, I shared the story with the nurse, Pauline. She listened intently to my saga.

In the hour long conversation, she convinced me that although We would all die one day, I would live long enough to see many of Brian's dreams come true. She convinced me that it was not necessary to spend $1700 that I did not have on a chicken coop for Brian. She convinced me that these feelings of sadness and doom would pass and that I would experience happier days. Because of Pauline, Brian never did get his chicken coop and I never went $1700 in debt and I have appreciated happier days. I will always remember the chicken coop story . . . but not so much about the chicken coop but because of Pauline. Pauline was herself going through treatment for pancreatic cancer. When I had been there on Monday for my own treatment, she finished her shift and then sat down in the treatment room for her own chemotherapy. Pauline died two months after this phone call. She lived and gave of herself right to the end. She is my role model for living and dying. Rest in Peace Pauline.